MEMOIR OF AN
ACCIDENTAL ETHICIST

MEMOIR OF AN
ACCIDENTAL ETHICIST

On medical ethics, medical misconduct and challenges for the medical profession

KERRY J. BREEN

AUSTRALIAN SCHOLARLY

© Kerry J. Breen 2018

First published 2018 by
Australian Scholarly Publishing Pty Ltd

7 Lt Lothian St Nth, North Melbourne, Vic 3051

Tel: 03 9329 6963 / Fax: 03 9329 5452
enquiry@scholarly.info / www.scholarly.info

ISBN 978-1-925801-22-4

Cover design: Wayne Saunders
Cover: Hippocratic Oath in Greek. From Vatican Manuscript Urbinus 64, folio 116. William Henry Samuel Jones, *The Doctor's Oath,* 1924

To the memory of
Greg Fournier-Breen
1975–2017

CONTENTS

ACKNOWLEDGEMENTS

A large number of mentors, role models and colleagues assisted me in my professional development over my career and many, but not all, are identified throughout this book. Hopefully my gratitude to these people is evident in what I have written. In addition, several colleagues and friends took the time to carefully read and critique all or parts of drafts of my manuscript, making numerous helpful suggestions and occasional corrections. They included Katrina Watson, Bernadette Tobin, Colin Thomson, Chris Cordner, Stephen Cordner, David Cade, James King, Laurie Geffen, David Weisbrot and Ron Brent. In addition respected biographer, Brenda Niall, read and helpfully commented on my text and provided sage advice. To all these people I am deeply grateful. Permission to use certain material was generously provided by the Medical Journal of Australia. I also wish to thank Nick Walker and his team at Australian Scholarly Publishing for their highly professional and timely assistance and advice.

PROLOGUE

A little while back, I was interviewed by a medical colleague for an oral history project on the topic of the Medical Practitioners Board of Victoria. I had known this colleague for many years and we had served together on the Board for a short time. Early in the interview, he asked me when and where I had obtained my training in medical ethics. I was so surprised by this question that my responses to his other inquiries over the next few minutes were barely intelligible. Running through my mind was the notion of 'if he does not know that I have had no formal training in medical ethics, what on earth do others who know me less well think?'

Later I had time to reflect on the brief interchange and could understand why my colleague had assumed that I had some training in medical ethics. I remained concerned that other doctors had made the same assumption and that in effect I might be seen to be holding myself out to be something that I wasn't. My reflections also had me thinking about a closely related aspect of my interest in medical ethics, a notion that had emerged slowly through my involvement in the subject. This was my desire to encourage as many doctors as possible to engage in debates around medical ethics and never to be intimidated by lack of formal training in ethics nor be put off by the use of ethical jargon and sophisticated terminology by those doctors and others, including those in the new field of bioethics, who have had such formal training.

My initial aims in writing this memoir were two-fold. One was to set the record straight about how I have never had any training in medical ethics. Indeed, as the record of how I became interested in and eventually passably knowledgeable about medical ethics will reveal, I might be called an 'accidental ethicist'. A second aim was to continue in my quest to make all doctors comfortable about contributing to discussions around medical ethics, using that term in its broadest sense.

However, as I wrote the story, it gradually became clear to me that I was also creating a partial history of the evolution of many aspects of the regulation of the medical profession over the last four decades. Thus, I have delved into some thorny ethical issues for the profession, including problematic relations with drug companies, how to best help doctors who become unwell and possibly unfit to practise, particular forms of professional misconduct including sexual misconduct and misconduct in undertaking research, and the pros and cons of the national scheme to regulate the medical profession. As high ethical standards are regarded nowadays as a key hallmark of a 'good doctor', late in the evolution of my story I was prompted to add a chapter about what I think are the qualities that are needed to make a good doctor.

Hopefully, as well as addressing my two original aims, my memoir might also make interesting reading for those wishing to know more about what goes on behind the scenes in medical ethics, medical regulation, research misconduct, and issues around the health and well-being of doctors. Reading it might even attract senior doctors in busy clinical practice to give their time to sit on a medical board or a medical tribunal where clinical experience, wisdom, and some interest in or knowledge of professionalism, medical ethics and medical law is of relevance and value.

One of the barriers to doctors feeling comfortable engaging in discussion and debate about ethical issues or about ethical aspects of medical care is a fear of being intimidated by those who have expertise in ethics, as if ethics is some magical realm only inhabited by experts. I know that there was a time when I felt intimidated in this manner. My self-confidence grew slowly but was especially bolstered when a philosopher/ethicist colleague provided a very simple definition of what ethics is all about. That definition, elaborated slightly here, is as follows: 'Ethics and ethical codes can be seen as an accumulation of values and principles that address questions of what is good or bad in human affairs. Ethics searches for reasons for acting or refraining from acting; for approving or not approving conduct; for believing or denying something about virtuous or vicious conduct or good or evil rules'. So when you are debating an ethical issue in clinical medicine, all you are doing is participating in a process of trying to make a decision as to what is the best or the right thing to do after considering all the relevant circumstances or competing interests. When discussing or thinking about problems faced in clinical practice, doctors are frequently doing just this without realising it. Indeed, in his 1983 book *The Unmasking of Medicine*, Professor Ian Kennedy wrote that 'each diagnosis of illness is an ethical decision'.[*]

---

[*] Kennedy, I, *The Unmasking of Medicine*, revised edn., London: Granada, 1983.

This account is mostly about my experiences. These include a few negative experiences in my relationships with individuals. To avoid hurting people through my description of some of these relationships, I have chosen in almost every instance not to identify the people involved. I do not think that anyone acted other than in good will and a belief that they were trying to do the right thing. Although I disagreed with them and in places I give my reasons why, I have no wish to harm their reputations. On the other hand, I happily name the many excellent people with whom I have worked over the years and who deserve much praise, usually for their work behind the scenes, work that was primarily for the broader benefit of our community and was often unremunerated or only partly remunerated.

I describe numerous occasions where I was the beneficiary of serendipity. Indeed even my decision to enrol to study to become a doctor involved serendipity. Serendipitous or chance opportunities need to be taken of course. This is more likely to happen where one is willing to take on new tasks and, to a degree, has a prepared state of mind.

Chapter 1

AN UNLIKELY MEDICAL STUDENT

A bush childhood

In choosing a career as a doctor, chance far outweighed logic and I was very fortunate that I found myself reasonably well-suited to many of the tasks of being a doctor. My life story in a nutshell before I became a doctor is as follows. I was born in the Bright Bush Nursing Hospital in north-eastern Victoria in 1941. My father was a primary school teacher. His parents were subsistence farmers near St Arnaud where he was born, the fourth of eleven children. A second generation Australian, he was of totally Irish descent (his mother was a Murphy). My mother, née Zeven, was three-quarter Irish and one quarter Dutch by descent. She was one of four children and was born and raised in the Essendon area in Melbourne. A few months before I was born, my parents, with my older brother and sister, had moved from Ocean Grove to Freeburgh, six miles south of Bright in the Ovens Valley on the road to Harrietville. The primary school at Freeburgh, first opened in 1865, had once enrolled around one hundred pupils in the days of the Victorian gold rush but now was a single room solo teacher school with twenty or less pupils who lived within a mile or two of the school. My father by then was quite accustomed to solo teacher primary schools having taught at Ocean Grove with an enrolment of around twenty-five pupils and before that at smaller schools in Lubeck and Coromby in the Wimmera and earlier, before he married, at Arawata in Gippsland.

At Freeburgh, there was ongoing evidence of the gold rush era with a working gold dredge near to the school on the plain of the Ovens Valley and dangerous disused mine tunnels in the adjacent hills. We lived in the teacher's residence next to the school. This was a simple three bedroom timber house without running water, heating, electricity or sewerage. We used tank water in which we often found 'wrigglers' or the larvae of mosquitoes. A wood stove was used for cooking. The only means for cooling food was a Coolgardie safe, a simple evaporative device, hung outdoors. Our lighting was with kerosene lamps, or by candlelight if you wanted to read in bed. We did not own a radio until I was about six years old. It was powered by a car battery which needed to be regularly taken into Bright to be recharged. Radio reception in the valley was only possible at night and even then, the only strong signal came from the ABC station, 2CO, in Corowa in New South Wales. In the absence of sewerage or septic tanks, the teacher's duties included regularly burying the pan contents not only of our outdoor dunny but also of the boys' and girls' toilets in the school yard.

Our nearest neighbour, Mrs Flynn, lived half a mile away where she ran the Freeburgh Post Office from a room in the front of her home. Freeburgh had no shops, hotel or any businesses. All food and other supplies came from Bright.

We did not have a car so once a week my mother took the bus that ran from Harrietville into Bright to shop. Some of our time at Freeburgh was during World War II but we were as far away from the war as was possible. My mother's shopping was affected by war-time rationing. My father's occupation was protected so he was not obliged to join several of his brothers who served in the Army. He spent at least one summer vacation working in a munitions factory in Melbourne.

I commenced school at a young age as I was allowed to spend the day in school from the age of three and a half. This was against Education Department rules. A photo from that year, 1945, shows that enrolment had dropped to eleven pupils, including six from one family. Apart from a year of correspondence school when I was seven and a year of riding a bike six miles and back every day to a larger school in Bright when I was eight, my teacher for my entire primary education was my father. Schooling by correspondence was needed because the school at Freeburgh was closed when the enrolment dropped below seven pupils. For the next two years, the Education Department kept us living in the teacher's residence at Freeburgh while my father was sent to teach at another small school at Ovens near Myrtleford. He rode his bicycle to Bright early on Monday mornings, took the train to Myrtleford and stayed in the Ovens Hotel, returning home on Friday evenings. The Ovens Hotel may have been where his difficulties with alcohol began.

My mother also played a role in my primary education. She supervised my year of correspondence learning and was a teacher's aide at a couple of my primary schools. In that era the Education Department encouraged the wives of teachers in remote areas to work part-time in schools under the official title of 'sewing mistress', but in reality my mother did much more than this and could be more accurately called a teacher's aide. Later, in the 1960s, she taught classes of seventy pupils in a large suburban Catholic primary school in Melbourne, although she never gained formal qualifications as a teacher. Unusual at the time for women, she had completed her Leaving Certificate which was as far as secondary education then went. With the hindsight of a lifetime, I suspect now that she was at least as intelligent as my father and possibly more so.

My father was progressive in his ideas about teaching. He opposed corporal punishment both at school and in the home. He only firmly smacked me once as a child but, even today, I recognise that I deserved it. I had admired the woodchoppers at the Bright Agricultural Show and as a seven-year-old took to practising with our axe on the young eucalypts beyond the school yard fence. Becoming bored with the softness of the green eucalypts, I found a hard wood post to practise on and was halfway through it when my father found me. I had selected for my practice one of the two netball posts in the school grounds!

My father was keen that his pupils were exposed to Australian authors as much as possible. For several years at Freeburgh, he wrote to the Education Department each year requesting funds for a small library for the school. The funding finally was granted and he purchased one hundred or so books, mostly authored by Australians. Not long after the arrival of this collection the school was officially closed. My father then asked the Department what he should do with the new 'library'. He was instructed to take care of it

4

until further notice. That notice never came and some of the collection is still held by my younger sister, a retired librarian. When we left Freeburgh, we also took the tall timber cupboard in which the books were kept. Ten years later, I took the shelves out of the cupboard and turned it into a rather slim wardrobe for a bungalow that I shared with my older brother.

My father disliked and resented the men who gave up teaching to become school inspectors. He could not understand why they would give up the joys of teaching. We had a dog at Freeburgh, a lovely part-Kelpie black mongrel, which rarely showed any inclination to be aggressive towards strangers. His behaviour one day of grasping the school inspector by the heel as he approached the schoolyard gate made him even more loved by my father. My father was intolerant of bureaucrats, especially those employed by the Education Department. He was said to have written letters to the newspapers critical of the Department although I have never sighted the letters. I suspect that this was true as, based on the evidence of his teaching placements especially the one that followed Freeburgh and Ovens, he was not always well-treated by the Department.

While living conditions in Freeburgh were primitive by modern standards, it was a wonderful place for a childhood. As long as we stayed away from the old gold tunnels, we were free to roam the valley, including spending time watching the gold dredge. In the nine years that we lived there, the dredge, working around the clock six days per week, moved slowly up and down the Ovens Valley adjacent to the school. It turned the soil upside down leaving tailings of rock and sand. Environmentally it was disastrous. One spin off was the obligation on the owners to 'rehabilitate' the area and this was done by planting pine trees, thereby creating another industry in due course.

After school we had the entire well-grassed school playground to ourselves, although shared with the hens from our hen house. Next to the teacher's residence my father created a large vegetable garden. We also kept a cow in an adjacent paddock. It was my mother's task to milk our cow, named Judy, every morning and evening. In summer after school, Mum or Dad walked us through snake infested paddocks to swim in the clear waters of the Ovens River. Snakes were a hazard in the school playground. I don't know when snakes were first protected in Victoria. If they were protected in the 1940's, this was another bureaucratic rule that my father ignored. For the safety of his pupils, he preferred to kill any snakes found in the school grounds. I recall one summer ten or more dead snakes hanging on the wire fence that surrounded the playgrounds. Just behind the school grounds, where the foothills to the alps began, ran a small culvert diverting water from the Ovens River to the gold dredge. The culvert (we called it our 'ditch') became a place for fun and at times for successful fishing for trout, including the illegal method of leaving lines in overnight.

Outdoor activities dominated our lives. We used the school grounds for playing 'kick to kick' football and my older brother and sister built a rough court for tennis. My brother, six years older, allowed me at times to take part in his other activities, which included ferreting for rabbits, of plague proportions then. He also allowed me to use his air rifle. I was not allowed to use his 22-gauge rifle nor the powerful US army disposal automatic rifle that an unwise uncle sent him. The latter was accurate but so powerful that the target rabbit was not recognisable when shot. As a special treat, I was permitted one night to accompany a neighbour whose living was partly based on trapping rabbits and selling the skins to a Melbourne hat maker. I was amazed how, in the dark, she could unerringly locate the traps she had set the previous night. In summer, she picked wild blackberries (also present in plague proportions) and shipped these in four-gallon 'kerosene tins' to a Melbourne jam factory.

Not long before we left Freeburgh, my father had another experience that reinforced his negative view of bureaucrats. The outdoor laundry building at the teacher's residence was in a bad state of disrepair when my family arrived in 1941 and he had repeatedly requisitioned its replacement. A new laundry was finally built just a few months before we left and nearly two years after the school was closed. He explained to me at the time that although his request had to be made via the Education Department, the work was authorised by the Public Works Department and undertaken, after a successful tender, by a local builder, probably based in Wangaratta. The fact that the school was closed would have been carefully ignored by the builder.

Further into the bush

Our time in Freeburgh ended when I was nine. In 1950, the Education Department posted my father to Glen Valley. Glen Valley then was probably the smallest, highest, coldest and most isolated village in Victoria, situated on a narrow dangerous unsealed road part way between Omeo and Mitta

Mitta. The house provided was timber and had never had an external coat of paint. As at Freeburgh, there was no power, running water or septic tank. There was a small general store across the road from us and a nearby tiny single room wooden building used by a butcher who came from Omeo once a week. The school was again a single classroom with a solo teacher, assisted by the part-time 'sewing mistress', my mother. The school was half a mile from our house. Three miles further up the road towards Mitta Mitta stood the Glen Wills Hotel. Nearby Mt Wills had been the site of a gold rush at the turn of the century and at one point was a tent 'city' of seven thousand people. Although Glen Wills and Glen Valley still appear on maps, the Glen Valley school has been converted into a private house while the Glen Wills hotel and the house we lived in no longer exist.

In 1950 there was still a working gold mine, the Maude and Yellow mine, at Glen Valley. Soon after we arrived, a young accountant, Adrian Black, came from Melbourne to manage the mine. He brought with him his wife, Patricia, and their baby boy. They were our neighbours although neighbour was a relative term as they lived half a mile away on the other side of the narrow valley. They became close friends of our family and remained so for the rest of their lives. There were a number of reasons for the closeness including isolation, a common religion, similar interests and level of education, and for my father and the young accountant, a liking to spend Friday evenings and most of Saturday at the Glen Wills Hotel. With this new family's arrival, the Catholic priest in Omeo was prevailed upon to come once a month to say Mass in the Black's lounge room. I made my first communion in their home and Patricia Black took the communion preparation class of my younger sister and I and two other local children for this event.

Glen Valley was truly isolated. Newspapers took two days to arrive. My older brother and sister, now staying with relatives in Melbourne for their secondary schooling, also took two days if they came home for the school holidays. Their trip involved a train to Bairnsdale and a bus to Omeo where they stayed in a hotel for the night before next day taking the small bus that ran from Omeo to Mitta Mitta. For the first summer holidays in Glen Valley, they brought the measles home with them and all four of us were ill with measles, seriatim, in a fashion that filled the entire six weeks. My older sister was very seriously ill. We had no access to a doctor. Fortunately, Patricia Black had only recently completed her nursing training at St Vincent's Hospital in Melbourne. She moved into our house for a few nights to help my mother care for my sister, a generous act that bound the two mothers in friendship for the rest of their lives.

I was now in Grade 4 in a class of four pupils. My school report, completed and signed by my father, placed me first in the class. From Glen Valley, I had my first publication, a letter in the junior section of Argus newspaper extolling the virtues of life in the country.[*] We were only at Glen Valley for fifteen or so months and my recollections of that school experience are limited. I do recall that we went one day to Swifts Creek for the annual district school athletics carnival. The transport used for this 160-kilometre round trip was a large tip truck from the Maude and Yellow mine with most of the thirty or so school children sitting on rugs in the open

---

[*] https://trove.nla.gov.au/newspaper/article/23017209?searchTerm=kerry%20breen&searchLimits=l-title=13.

tray of the truck. Parts of the unsealed road to Omeo were very narrow with precipitous drops into steep valleys. The trip back that evening must have been a tense one for the driver.

The one winter we were at Glen Valley we had some heavy snowfalls, when we walked to school in gumboots. There were no local winter sports but I did construct my own toboggan, which worked in a fashion. Walking in fresh snow for the first time was a strange experience. The snow seemed to make the whole valley quieter and also let you walk much more quietly. I was allowed to roam where I wished and one weekend I came across a 'family' of emus also walking in the snow not far from where I was standing. They were unperturbed by my presence. Other wild life commonly encountered included kangaroos and lyrebirds.

In 1951, part way through the year, we moved closer to Melbourne as my father was sent to teach at Yarrambat, again a single room school. I completed my primary schooling there. For my secondary education I attended Eltham High School for two years, travelling each day from Yarrambat by school bus. This was followed by four years as a boarder at Assumption College, Kilmore. Boarding only happened by chance as we had moved yet again, now to Greenvale, another single room school. At Greenvale we lived in a newly built teacher's residence where for the first time we had electricity and an indoor toilet. This was 1955. There was no easy public transport to the nearest boys' school. The choice of Kilmore was never in question as my father and some of his brothers had attended the college when their parents moved from the farm at St Arnaud to run a general store at Kilmore. My father had long before taught me the

Assumption College war-cry so in one small aspect I was prepared for this experience! These four years were the only formal Catholic education that I received.

From an educational viewpoint I thrived at boarding school. In Year 10, I had a stimulating English teacher, a Marist brother, Brother Marius Woulfe, who selected me as a member of a three-person debating team. This simple experience led me to telling people that I thought that I might become a lawyer. By now, my older brother and sister were at university and this, together with parental expectations, made it almost automatic that I too would seek to attend university. The idea of becoming a doctor had never entered my head and the position of careers adviser did not then exist. My family had no relatives or friends who were doctors and I had had virtually no experience of being sufficiently ill to need a doctor. Then chance intervened again.

How I chose to study medicine

In the summer holiday before our matriculation year (Year 12), my best friend at school invited me to stay with his family in Maryborough in north-west Victoria for two weeks. His father was a general practitioner. I only met him at the dinner table each evening and did not visit his practice. However, through meeting him, in my young and naïve mind I perceived that doctors were normal people and thus I felt that I too could become a doctor! At the end of the year, I applied to enrol in the MBBS course at the University of Melbourne and was accepted. The three preclinical years were a hard slog of learning enormous amounts of anatomy, physiology, biochemistry and other material by heart. The three clinical years at St Vincent's Hospital with stints at the Royal Children's and Royal Women's Hospitals were much more enjoyable. Over time I realised that fortunately I was well suited to most of the roles expected of doctors. Thus I never regretted this career choice.

While there was nothing in my childhood environment that might explain my wish to become a doctor, in hindsight I can see influences from my childhood that had an impact on where my career as a doctor took me. As an adult, I experienced intense discomfort with confrontation and disagreement, leading me to be a natural peacemaker and facilitator. As already hinted at, my father had an alcohol problem which gradually worsened when I was still a young boy. When drunk, he was noisy and obstreperous and sometimes threatened my mother with violence. I learned as a young boy that he tempered this behaviour if I was present. As an eleven-year-old, I once moved to stand between my father and my mother when he was threatening her with a carving knife. Living with and learning to cope with the anxiety that I felt for my mother undoubtedly influenced the person (and doctor) that I became. Being away from this environment at boarding school undoubtedly allowed my academic performance to improve, giving me the opportunity to attend university.

My rural upbringing and a less affluent childhood than many of my peers made it easy for me to identify with less well-off people, with underdogs, and with anyone who had experienced a rural childhood. Having seen my father's career adversely affected by his willingness to publicly criticise the education bureaucracy (and school inspectors, privately) and to openly express his political views, I realised that it was wiser to generally conceal my political views, which, like my parents', were left of centre.

My parents were avid readers and my father dabbled in verse and prose, some of which was published. Children's books were not well provided for at the public library in Bright so I was reading (by candlelight) authors such as J B Priestley and Compton McKenzie at the age of nine. A love of literature and writing followed. In the medical course that I undertook, two essential qualities for good examination results were a good memory and, as most exams involved writing essays, a capacity to write quickly and clearly. My childhood had prepared me well for this.

I entered the medical course feeling that most of my contemporaries who had attended large Melbourne schools were all smarter and better educated than I. I was totally unaware of where I stood. I was ignorant of the fact that having won a Victorian Junior Government Scholarship in Year 9 placed me quite well. We were told that one in five would fail the first year of the medical course. Knowing that failure would lead to loss of my Commonwealth Scholarship (and force me out of the course) motivated me to study very hard. Luckily, I was living at home, now in North Essendon, with few distractions. I was very surprised at my good results in first year. From that time on, I continued to study hard to maintain these results. Overconfidence was unlikely to ever be a big problem for me.

I was never distracted through involvement in extracurricular activities at the University of Melbourne. I regretted that later but at the time, shyness, lack of confidence, and the need to take on part-time work to support myself, to have enough money for petrol for my 1939 model Vauxhall tourer car, and to provide for a limited social life, prevented such involvement. I did not have to pay board to my parents, a debt that, through their relatively premature deaths, I feel that I never repaid. We only spent the first three of the six years of the course on the university campus. After that, our lives as clinical students were very different, and the academic year was much longer. The latter had an impact on the nature of the part-time work that I sought but this proved to be educationally relevant.

In the first three years of the course, we were free of classes on Saturday mornings and I worked as a sales assistant in a local men's wear shop each Saturday until midday. During the long summer vacations of three months, I took on, at different times, various roles including office clerk, factory assembly worker, postman, gardener, sign writer and painter, and mortuary attendant at a public hospital. In fourth year of the course, I was allocated to the clinical school at St Vincent's Hospital where the academic year began at the end of January, limiting the weeks available in summer for full-time work. I needed to find a regular part-time position that was compatible with my time-table at St Vincent's, where mostly we were free at around 4.00 pm each day. Luckily, I found work as a barman at the late Peter Poynton's Carlton Club Hotel in Grattan St where I worked from 4.30 to 7.00 pm on weekdays and all day on Saturdays. These were the days when hotels closed at 6.00 pm. Peter was a generous employer and had no difficulty with me arriving late when afternoon lectures were occasionally scheduled from 4.00 to 5.00 pm. I worked for him throughout 1962 and 1963 but had to relinquish the job when I went to live in as a student at the

Royal Women's Hospital for the last ten weeks of 1963. The barman role was my longest and the most educational that I took on. I learnt more about alcohol and alcoholism in my two years in that job than during the medical course.

Early years as a doctor

The sixth year of the course finally was over we graduated and found work as junior medical residents, at a time when 'resident' meant exactly that. We lived at the hospital and had two evenings off per week from 6.00 pm until midnight. In choosing my rotations at St Vincent's, serendipity again came to my aid. I had made up my mind to apply to spend my three months on a medical ward with a visiting physician, Dr John Cahill, whom I greatly admired. However, on the way to lodge my application form, I encountered a friend from my boarding school, Dr Jack Kennedy, who had graduated a year ahead of me. He asked me about my choices and rapidly convinced me that I should instead apply to spend three months in the university academic department of medicine headed by Professor Carl de Gruchy. This was a good decision as this became my first rotation and I spent it under the guidance of a very thoughtful and thorough physician, Dr Albert Baikie, supported by his outstanding registrar, Dr John Cade (jnr). In my second year as a resident, on John Cade's advice, I spent three months working under cardiac surgeon, John Clarebrough, who later became one of my strongest supporters. He too was a very good role model in that he clearly respected his patients and would take infinite time to talk with patients and their families. Looking back, these mentors and role models were highly ethical in every aspect of their professional lives – but this was never remarked upon then and they themselves would not have given the matter any thought. If they thought about it at all, they would have seen themselves as simply striving to be good doctors.

Another powerful influence on my development but one that is difficult to measure was the presence of the Sisters of Charity who owned and ran St Vincent's. In the 1960s, there was a nun who was also a trained nurse in charge of every ward and they were present for most of the daytime hours. The philosophy of the hospital from its opening in 1893 was to care for the poor who were ill. This philosophy permeated the place, resulting in respect for every patient who entered its doors. I read more recently the views of an American commentator who suggested that the ethos and environment created in a hospital run by people who are not doctors is remarkably different to a hospital run by doctors for doctors. My long experience at St Vincent's Hospital supports that view. Any doctor who did not embrace the caring philosophy of the hospital would not be on the staff for long.

As a medical student at the University of Melbourne and at St Vincent's Hospital between 1959 and 1964, I cannot recall at any point being exposed to lectures, discussions, or other forms of teaching about medical ethics, so I am unable to claim even the most basic grounding in this subject. After graduation, I chose to train as a specialist physician, becoming qualified in general internal medicine and in gastroenterology. This involved four years as a resident medical officer and registrar at St Vincent's Hospital in Melbourne, eighteen months at the Royal Prince Alfred

Hospital in Sydney and two years at Vanderbilt University Medical School in the USA. While I learned an enormous amount in those years and fortunately was exposed to some outstanding role models (physicians and surgeons), again ethical issues were not formally part of my training or that exposure. I sat for and passed the examinations for membership of the Royal Australasian College of Physicians in Brisbane in 1968 and medical ethics was not part of the curriculum for those examinations.

In 1972, on my return from the USA, I took up my first senior clinical appointment at St Vincent's Hospital, Melbourne, as an honorary outpatient physician, followed by two years as a senior lecturer in the University of Melbourne academic Department of Medicine, also at St Vincent's Hospital. In 1975, I took on a full-time position as a staff gastroenterologist at the same hospital but maintained my role as a physician in general medicine, running an outpatient clinic twice per week. In 1978, I was appointed the inaugural Director of the Gastroenterology Unit at St Vincent's. My roles in both general medicine and gastroenterology were to continue until 1986, when I gave up my work as a general physician.

Once again despite my exposure to a broad range of medicine, I do not recall any participation in discussions of ethical matters during these years. In 1982, St Vincent's Hospital appointed the late Dr Nicholas Tonti-Filippini as its part-time hospital ethicist but, perhaps because he was not medically qualified, his appointment seemed to have little or no impact on most of the clinicians at that hospital. This role at St Vincent's Hospital has been stated to be the first appointment of a hospital ethicist in Australia. At the time of his appointment, Tonti-Filippini was a relatively new graduate who had studied in Professor Peter Singer's department at Monash University and had not then completed his PhD in ethics. His appointment to a newly created position where he had to face the scepticism of experienced clinicians probably made this a very difficult role for him. I later developed a great respect for his intellect. He moved on to other roles and became a prominent bioethicist and national figure.

My full-time staff appointment came with an entitlement to sabbatical leave which I first took from December 1980, spending six months working with some outstanding liver specialists in the hepatology department at Beaujön Hospital in Paris. In late 1981, a few months after my return to Melbourne, I received a letter which was to be a turning point in my career and in hindsight marked the beginning of my involvement in ethical issues in medicine. Prior to opening that letter, if anyone had asked me what my plans were for the next 15 to 20 years, I am sure I would have said that I was going to concentrate on my career as a clinician-teacher and researcher in gastroenterology and remain involved in practising general medicine. I recall that in the back of my mind, I was concerned that it would be undesirable for St Vincent's Hospital, and possibly for me, that I remain Director of the Gastroenterology service for too long and that I needed to keep an open mind about other career options.

Chapter 2

A LETTER AND ITS CONSEQUENCES

Appointment to the Medical Board

The 1981 letter was from Mr Bill Borthwick, then the Minister for Health in Victoria, informing me that I had been appointed to the Medical Board of Victoria and that I could expect to be contacted by the Board President, Dr Bernard Neal, about my duties. To say that I was surprised by the letter is definitely an understatement. I had not applied for appointment, I had not been approached by anyone about it, and indeed I had almost forgotten that the Medical Board existed. I clearly recalled presenting myself to the Medical Board offices along with all the other new medical graduates in late December 1964 to be registered. We paid ten guineas and were told we were registered for life. Some of my contemporaries, driven by impecuniousness and possessing more self-confidence than I, headed off immediately to take up two to three-week locum positions in urban or rural general practice before commencing as junior medical residents in their various hospitals early in January 1965. After that initial contact, the Medical Board remained invisible to most medical graduates.

In 1970, the Victorian Parliament passed a new *Medical Practitioners Act*. As I recall, this had only two noticeable effects: registration as a doctor now became subject to annual renewal (the fees for which went into consolidated revenue) and the junior resident medical officer year became the intern year, subject to provisional registration. This meant that general practice locum work was no longer possible until full registration was granted at the end of a satisfactory intern year. The Medical Board continued to remain invisible; it was not obliged to produce and circulate an annual report, it issued no newsletters to the profession, its disciplinary hearings were held behind closed doors and if a doctor's registration was suspended or cancelled, this news was well-concealed in the *Government Gazette*, a weekly publication that was read by few journalists and no doctors.

So, I had really no idea what the Board did and even less idea of how much work would be involved. Nevertheless, the letter from the Minister created for me a sense of obligation and public duty. In addition, I became aware that one of my mentors and supporters at St Vincent's Hospital, cardiac surgeon, Dr John Clarebrough, was a member of the Board and I felt that I might be letting him down if I rejected the appointment. I thus awaited a call from Dr Neal. By accepting that appointment, I was changing the direction of much of the rest of my career but I only became aware of that many years later.

Readers who are aware of the more complex processes (including advertisement, written applications, interviews and reference checks) now involved in appointments to the Medical Board may have difficulty believing this account of my appointment but this is exactly as it happened. I was never told how or why my name was put forward to the Minister but I did become aware that in that era it was common for the Minister to seek the advice of the relevant registration board if a vacancy occurred. The fact that I was known to two members of the Board, namely John Clarebrough and Prince Henry's Hospital-based general physician and gastroenterologist, Dr Harry Garlick, may have been what led to my appointment. Incidentally, like medical registration in the 1960s, appointment to the Medical Board in the 1980s seemed to have no time limits. This was not strictly true as the Act stated that membership was for three years but was renewable indefinitely. John Clarebrough served for 25 years, Harry Garlick for 19 years and I also stayed for 19 years.

My first Board meeting was an unusual one in that its sole purpose was to register new graduates from one of our medical schools (the University of Melbourne or Monash University) ahead of their intern year. I had received no induction into Board membership and no documentation other than a copy of the *Medical Practitioners Act*. This of course contained little that I could use to guide me in the task of meeting and 'signing up' my share of the new graduates. I did overhear the words being used by the Board members sitting on either side of me around the board table so I managed to get through the long process, hopefully not alerting the new graduates that I knew as little as they did about the workings of the Medical Board! The only message of real value was to advise each new registrant to keep the Board informed of their current mailing address because failure to receive the notice to renew registration each year was by far the commonest reason for doctors' names being removed from the Register.

I soon found that the Board normally met every second week at 3.30 pm on a Thursday to deal with the business before it. The meetings then were held in the Old Treasury Building in Spring Street, not too far for me to get to readily from St Vincent's Hospital. At my first routine meeting of the Board, the President formally welcomed me as a new member with a few words, the only ones of which I now recall were 'welcome to the crème de la crème', words which hinted at how some members possibly saw their status. Later I was to become aware that Dr Neal had been appointed President just one year earlier and that his appointment had come as some surprise to fellow Board members who had felt that longer serving member, Dr Harry Garlick, would be favoured by the Minister. If this was also felt by Dr Garlick, he gave no hint of it in his energetic embrace of the role of Deputy President.

The Board totalled nine members, all doctors, and only one a woman. Four of the nine had served at some point as president of the Victorian Branch of the Australian Medical Association, which also told me a little about how previous health ministers had made these appointments. One board member was also serving as President of the Medical Defence Association of Victoria. The Medical Defence Association of Victoria provided assistance and indemnity for doctors facing allegations of negligence in the civil courts or allegations of misconduct before the Medical Board. At that time, although it was not the only such body in Victoria, it was estimated to cover approximately 80% of Victorian doctors. His appointment to the Medical Board involved a conflict of interest about which nobody seemed concerned.

St Vincent's Hospital generously permitted me to take time away from my full-time staff position to sit on the Board. While preparation for Board meetings and the drafting of letters and other documents were done in my own time, the Board appointment involved a half a day's absence every fortnight and occasional absences for disciplinary hearings. My involvement in the latter was infrequent in the first ten years. Thus I continued to meet all my clinical, teaching and administrative commitments as a gastroenterologist and general physician while I served on the Medical Board. This remained so until 1996 when I took long-service leave from St Vincent's. Although my ongoing clinical experience underpinned my role as a Board member, that clinical experience was little different to that of any other clinician and there seems no need to dwell on that aspect of my career in this story.

The health ministers over the years were aware of the desirability of having a broad spectrum of clinical backgrounds at the Medical Board table. When I was appointed, the membership included two general practitioners, two physicians, two surgeons, a psychiatrist/ administrator, an obstetrician and a paediatric physician (the President). All members other than the obstetrician were aged over sixty and I had just turned forty. It is another understatement to say that I felt ill-equipped and inexperienced for this new role. It was to be a rapid learning curve.

The Board was supported by a staff of five people, public servants seconded from various government departments.

One of these was more senior and served as the Registrar to the Board. The Medical Board had no say in these appointments and had to accept the staff it was allocated. Shortly after my appointment, this process led to a new Registrar who had until recently worked in the liquor licensing section of government. He had joined the public service having completed year eleven at a country high school. While this background seemed to me to be less than ideal, he proved to be a very hard-working individual who served the interests of the community, the profession and the Board extremely well and was still the Board Registrar nineteen years later. Another staff member was a secretary/typist who was the quickest and most accurate typist I have ever had the pleasure to work with. She too outlasted my time with the Medical Board.

The work of the Medical Board

The Board's major work was to receive, assess and deal with complaints made against doctors. It also dealt each fortnight with applications for registration and with notifications about doctors admitted to psychiatric hospitals. Complaints, mostly from patients or their relatives, but also at times from insurance companies and government agencies frustrated at the tardiness of doctors asked to provide medical reports, were received in writing and were handled by the Board 'on the papers'. No investigations were conducted and complainants and doctors were never interviewed by Board members or staff. What amounted to a form of investigation was to send the letter of complaint to the doctor concerned and ask for a written response. That response was then considered by the full Board and a decision taken as to the outcome. Other than in the most egregious situations, the commonest outcome was that the explanation provided by the doctor was accepted by the Board and a brief letter was sent to the complainant stating that no action would be taken. This approach changed a little during my first years on the Board in that, if deemed appropriate, the Board would include advice in its correspondence to the doctor that implied some criticism and make suggestions as to how such a complaint might have been avoided.

The lack of a public profile of the Medical Board created another problem. It was not uncommon that patients, not knowing to whom to complain (and note that at this time, the Health Services Commissioner role was yet to be created), would lodge their complaint with the Victorian branch of the Australian Medical Association (AMA Victoria), or occasionally with one of the medical colleges. It was clear that these pathways were generally a 'brick wall' for patients. If the doctor was a member of AMA Victoria, a perfunctory investigation universally found in favour of the doctor. If the doctor was not a member of the AMA (and a majority were not), the patient was simply informed that this was the case and that the AMA could not deal with the complaint. Neither the AMA nor the relevant medical college bothered to inform the complainant of the existence of the Medical Board.

Less commonly the Medical Board received complaints that were sufficiently serious that action was unavoidable. When this was the case, the Board used its powers to hold disciplinary inquiries. Under the *Medical Practitioners*

Act 1970, the Board had the powers to hold two levels of inquiries. Under Section 16 of the Act a doctor could be brought before the Board if it was felt that the doctor had engaged in misconduct that might warrant a reprimand. Under Section 17 of the Act, an inquiry could be held into more serious allegations, i.e. those possibly warranting suspension or deregistration. In the former case, proceedings were relatively informal and the doctor was not permitted to have legal representation. In the latter case, the proceedings were quite formal, taking on a judicial tribunal format.

Section 17 hearings dealt with such matters as allegations of sexual misconduct, convictions for indictable (serious) offences, or the issuing of fraudulent medical certificates. In these cases, the Board referred the allegations and what evidence it had to the Victorian Government Solicitor's Office (VGSO) for preparation for a disciplinary inquiry before the Board. At such an inquiry, the doctor was legally represented and the VGSO briefed a barrister to appear as counsel-assisting to present the evidence to the Board and to examine and cross-examine witnesses before the Board. In sitting as disciplinary tribunal, the Board was required to have a quorum of five members, all of course doctors. As mentioned above, these inquiries were closed to the public and the media.

The 1970 *Medical Practitioners Act* provided that the Medical Board had the power to decide if a disciplinary hearing should be open or closed. By long unquestioned tradition, neither the Board nor doctors appearing before it were anxious that matters be heard in public. This was not challenged until a hearing into the conduct of Dr Geoffrey Edelsten in 1992. At a disciplinary inquiry into allegations of serious misconduct, viz. criminal conduct, Edelsten's legal team was instructed to request that the inquiry be open to the public. The Board agreed to this request. Each day a group of 15–20 members of the public sat in the inquiry room. Edelsten was doing the Board a favour, as the inquiry panel members soon realised that having the inquiry open to the public did not impinge on the proceedings in any significant manner.

The first such Section 17 disciplinary inquiry where I sat as a member of the Board forming the tribunal was in 1982 and involved allegations surrounding a suburban general practitioner who was using his practice as a type of small private hospital to undertake terminations of pregnancy. We recognised that, while he was acting within the law, the standard of medical care that he offered was questionable. Rather than trying to close his practice down and risk an appeal to the Supreme Court where the doctor might well win his case, the Board opted to place an order that he not undertake mid-term abortions.

A very distressing disciplinary inquiry

I participated in a more distressing Section 17 inquiry not long after that. An orthopaedic surgeon was alleged to have sexually abused several women who had attended him and in whom he made the diagnosis of coccydynia, or more simply, persistent pain in the coccyx. The doctor claimed that his treatment method which involved massage of the coccyx via the vagina was an effective and acceptable means of treatment. Six or seven women gave almost identical evidence that he had used his method to deliberately sexually stimulate them and at least one gave evidence that this 'treatment' had been followed by penetration with his erect penis. The experience of having to hear the testimony of several women speaking frankly about events that should never have happened to them was truly shocking. Their distress was great and very visible. Although these were events that were out of their control, a common theme in their evidence was deep shame that they had 'allowed' this to happen to them. While the inquiry was closed to the public and the media, the women gave their evidence to a panel of four male doctors and one female doctor. Both barristers were male. No support was offered to the women before or after the inquiry. It was to be several years before any such support was made available at Board inquiries.

To drag these women through the trauma and humiliation of being vigorously cross-examined in front of a predominantly male Board by a senior male barrister on behalf of the orthopaedic surgeon was an eye-opening introduction for me to the issue of sexual misconduct by doctors. Board members were unanimous that the charges were proven and at the end of the third day of the hearing the Board handed down an immediate decision to deregister the surgeon. Despite the powerful evidence of the women, I did not sleep well that night as I wondered about the board getting the decision wrong. To deregister a doctor is a serious matter. Late on the next day, we were informed that the surgeon had returned home, taken a gun and shot himself. He left a note for his family admitting his guilt. The doctor's suicide note eased my inexperienced mind about our decision but the suicide was clearly an enormous tragedy for his family. There are no winners in sexual misconduct cases. Like a number of Board experiences, this hearing had a profound effect on me. Later, I was able to channel this experience into seeking to improve the support provided to complainants in hearings of sexual misconduct allegations.

Most of the matters considered each fortnight by the Medical Board were far less serious than sexual misconduct. At first, I was quite surprised at how easily doctors could make 'mistakes' that led to complaints being made to the Board. Gradually I became aware that many of these mistakes were related to, or caused by, ignorance or lack of awareness of what I later called 'every day legal and ethical obligations' of doctors. I now cannot recall when it was that I began to use that phrase but it was also the point at which my interest in professional conduct and medical ethics accelerated.

To provide examples of common recurring complaints, four immediately come to mind; complaints from employers about back-dated medical certificates, notification from the Drugs and Poison section of the Health Department of breaches of the regulations surrounding dangerous (addictive) drugs, complaints from insurance companies about tardy provision of medical reports, and complaints from patients where a poor attitude to communication by the doctor appeared to be at the heart of the matter. No doctor can be completely immune from being the subject of a complaint and, after my appointment to the Board, I sensed myself taking even more care with communication and with medico-legal responsibilities in my own clinical work. In my years on the Board, only two serving members were ever the subject of complaint from a patient.

Looking back, I feel that the Board was at times quite

arbitrary in its decisions to hold inquiries under Section 16 of the Act. Although such inquiries were intended to be informal, they would have been experienced as quite threatening and stressful for any doctor asked to appear as the doctor faced the full Board membership. This was done not to intimidate the doctor but for the Board's convenience; i.e. so that the inquiry could form part of a routine board meeting. These did form part of many meetings, often prolonging the meetings until quite late in the evening. Soon our meetings were scheduled to begin at 2.00 pm, not at 3.30 pm, and often ran until 8.00 pm.

Only one Section 16 inquiry has stuck firmly in my mind. This was a sad event and possibly based in racism. The Board received at least two complaints from medical officers employed by two large manufacturing companies in Dandenong. The medical officers alleged that a number of local general practitioners had issued unjustified medical certificates certifying that many company staff were unfit to work. The certificates all covered the Vietnamese New Year (Tết, the most important celebration in Vietnamese culture) which that year fell on a weekday, the employees' names appeared to be Vietnamese, and the general practitioners were also apparently of Vietnamese origin.

Because of this pattern, it seemed to the Board that some or all of the certificates might not be based on convincing medical evidence of actual illness. Written responses from some of the general practitioners involved did not ease the Board's concerns. Instead of asking for the doctors' records or interviewing each doctor about the grounds for their certificates (some of which may indeed have been clinically justified), we decided to hold a 'group' Section 16 inquiry.

Thus, seven or eight doctors appeared collectively and sat in a row at one end of the large table around which we Board members were arranged. It must have been an intimidating experience for these doctors, all reasonably new to practice in Victoria. Fortunately, the Board decided not to take any action such as issuing a reprimand. Instead the President counselled the group about the seriousness that surrounds the issuing of sickness certificates and the care that must be taken in writing and attesting to what is a legal document. Thus, the Board never ascertained how many certificates were supplied in bad faith versus how many resulted from the patients being able to convincingly feign illness, or indeed how many patients were actually ill. My guess is that truly ill Vietnamese people in the district may have found it a little more difficult to get a sickness certificate over the ensuing months!

Under another Section of the *Medical Practitioners Act*, Section 18, the Board had the power to conduct inquiries into the health of doctors and their fitness to practice. Indeed, if the Board wished to suspend the registration of an impaired doctor, it was obliged to hold an inquiry. Such inquiries were held infrequently. There was an obligation under the Act for the medical superintendent of any mental hospital to notify the Board if a doctor was admitted to the hospital. Otherwise, unwell and impaired doctors were rarely notified to the Board, probably because of awareness of how stressful an appearance before a Board inquiry could be. The medical profession generally tried to deal with flagrant cases of impairment by the 'three wise men' approach, especially where it involved for example a senior surgeon continuing to operate when his skills were failing. This approach referred to the private and informal selection of three senior members of the profession to call on the doctor and suggest as forcefully as possible that the doctor retire from practice. I recall during my early years on the Board that there was much hand-wringing among senior Board members over an approach to one of Melbourne's best-known surgeons who was very reluctant to accept the advice of his peers to retire from operating.

In the 1990s, the Act was amended to make it less stressful for an allegedly impaired doctor to be handled by the Board. This amendment and other issues related to doctors' health subsequently became a major interest for me.

I also began to sense during my early years that the Medical Board, through dealing with these various cases, was accumulating a wealth of experience that should have been used to educate doctors and medical students. Eventually this became a reality through the publication of newsletters and bulletins to the profession and through the duty, imposed by government, that the Board produce an annual report to Parliament.

A very effective chairman

Bernard Neal was a very effective chair of Board proceedings, although his approach at times prolonged meetings, irking some members. I learned a lot about good chairmanship through observing him. For any difficult or contentious topic, he took pains to ensure that every Board member was given time to make a contribution to the discussion. He rarely inserted his own views into the discussion at this point. Instead he summed up what he had heard and drew out what he thought was the conclusion that the Board was coming to. It was unusual for Board members to question that conclusion. Of course there were occasions where agreement was more difficult and where Neal would add his personal opinion. In such situations, sensing that agreement was unlikely, he would at times adjourn the debate until our next Board meeting, allowing members to 'sleep on the matter'. This technique worked remarkably well.

I was struck early on by the seeming absence on the part of most Board members in any interest in seeking to improve the processes of the Board, and by the members apparent lack of curiosity in how sister regulatory bodies interstate and overseas met their responsibilities. A notable exception was Deputy President, Dr Harry Garlick, and I found myself drawn to supporting his views and actions. Garlick in the mid-1980s funded his own travel to Canada and took the initiative to visit medical board equivalents (called 'colleges') in two large Canadian provinces. What he found surprised him and he returned to our Board with enthusiasm that we could do much better in Victoria.

Garlick noted in particular that the colleges he visited employed medically qualified staff to undertake investigations of complaints, had legally qualified members and community members on the committees or panels that determined the outcome of complaints, produced informative annual reports that were sent to all doctors and, in between annual reports, issued regular bulletins for the profession. He encouraged his fellow board members in Victoria to seek to emulate these practices.

Board members were indeed supportive of these ideas

but, looking back, I feel that collectively we did not lobby hard enough for change. There were enormous obstacles of course. These changes had resource implications. As annual renewal of registration fees went into the Government's general revenue, the Board had no money to spend on any initiative, such as employing medically qualified investigation staff or issuing bulletins. Adding legally qualified and lay or community members to the Medical Board required amendments to the *Medical Practitioners Act*, something that happened as frequently as the appearance of Halley's comet, unless pressure was applied to government. That pressure needed to come from the medical profession collectively, as represented by AMA Victoria. To bring the AMA leadership on board with ideas that might lead to higher annual registration renewal fees and to 'dilution' of the profession's control of the Medical Board through the addition of non-medical members was placed in the too hard basket.

By now at least, the Board was preparing a brief annual report to Parliament although there was no money to pay for this to be circulated to the profession. Via that report, every year for four or five years, the Board repeated its request that legal and lay members be added to the membership of the Board. This finally happened in 1991 with generally positive consequences to which I will return.

The Board had more success in convincing the Minister that we needed the appointment of a part-time medically qualified investigating officer. The Board was provided with the funds to do this in around 1988. As the most junior member of the Board, I had no role in making that appointment. I am unaware of who the applicants were but the Board chose the recently retired and long-serving Medical Secretary of AMA Victoria, Dr Bill Ryall. Ryall had previously worked in general practice so he was not lacking in clinical experience but he was towards the end of his career, was not physically well, and was steeped in the AMA method of 'resolving' complaints. All that was achieved through his appointment was that individual Board members were relieved of drafting letters to (generally unsuccessful) complainants. All complaints continued to be dealt with on the papers and no active investigations were undertaken.

I do not now recall if I expressed my disappointment. If I had, it is unlikely to have had any impact. I was involved in another of Harry Garlick's initiatives however. As already mentioned, I thought that the Medical Board was holding a mine of material that could be used to educate the medical profession. So, when Dr Garlick proposed that the Board should summarise some instructive cases in its annual report and seek to have copies of the report sent to all registered doctors, I strongly supported him. I then assisted him in writing anonymised reports of selected disciplinary inquiries (both Section 16 and Section 17 inquiries) that the Board had conducted to be added to the annual report. A new era was gradually emerging.

Chapter 3

THE PROFESSIONAL PRACTICE COURSE

A key turning point

Just as my choice of career and my later appointment to the Medical Board had strong elements of chance, so too did my next experience that further changed the direction of my career and catapulted me more clearly into the medical ethics arena. In around 1989 or thereabouts, I attended a luncheon to which were invited members of the Medical Board and a range of other people involved with aspects of the work of the Board. The luncheon was arranged by the Board member who was also President of the Medical Defence Association of Victoria.

I found myself sitting next to Professor Stephen Cordner, whom I had not previously met. Stephen had not long before taken up his appointment as the inaugural director of the Victorian Institute of Forensic Pathology (VIFP), later renamed the Victorian Institute of Forensic Medicine. The Institute forms a part of the Coroner's Court complex and its primary role is to perform autopsies to determine the cause of death, most critically where homicide is suspected. Although academically the VIFP was and still is part of Monash University Faculty of Medicine, at that time Stephen's Institute was also responsible for delivering an educational program in law and ethics for medical students not only from Monash University but also for medical students from the University of Melbourne. Anyone familiar with how crowded a medical curriculum can become will not be surprised to learn that Stephen told me of his concerns that the limited teaching that his department could provide to these medical students was unlikely to sustain them throughout their careers.

I was in a position to reinforce his concerns by describing my experience at the Medical Board, now extending to seven or eight years. As I explained to him, the Board was continually seeing doctors who were coming to attention through what I sensed was a lack of knowledge and awareness of ethical and legal principles that underlay good medical practice. We rapidly agreed that there was a problem and also agreed to meet again soon to discuss whether we might find a solution. This was to be the beginning of a long-term friendship and a very rewarding professional collaboration.

When we met a couple of weeks later, Stephen brought with him Professor Vernon Plueckhahn. Vernon had not long retired from an impressive career as a pathologist and forensic pathologist and had more spare time than did Stephen or me. He was an energetic person with excellent organisational skills that he enjoyed employing. Plueckhahn had been one of the driving forces behind the establishment of VIFP, an Australian first. He was a mentor of Stephen Cordner. He was also senior author, with Stephen as co-author, of a very good text book, *Ethics, Legal Medicine and Forensic Pathology*, published by Melbourne University

Press. We decided at the meeting that what was needed was a means of reinforcing and extending what medical students were taught at VIFP to the post-graduate level and that a short part-time course for young doctors might meet this need. Fellow medical board member, surgeon Ian McVey, also supported this endeavour.

To garner wider support for the idea, we assembled a broad-based program committee that included a nominee from the Health Department, the Medical Postgraduate Foundation of Victoria, Melbourne and Monash Medical Schools, AMA Victoria, the Association of Medical Directors of Victorian Hospitals, the Health Services Commissioner and the Medical Defence Association of Victoria. We decided that for the first year we would run the program on five consecutive Wednesday afternoons at the VIFP which had an excellent lecture theatre for this purpose. There were to be no registration fees and all speakers for the program would be asked to contribute on an honorary basis. VIFP underwrote what costs were entailed.

The committee agreed that the primary target for the program would be hospital medical officers (registrars) nearing the end of their clinical training and about to enter unsupervised medical practice. We hoped that we would be able to convince the teaching hospitals to grant leave to such staff for five afternoons over five weeks. We called our proposal the 'Professional Practice Program'. This title was borrowed from the Leo Cussen Centre for Law which ran a course by this name designed to equip new law graduates with the skills needed to enter legal practice. In recommending this name, it did not cross my mind until much later that we were trying then to teach what twenty-five years afterwards became known in medical circles as 'medical professionalism'.

In planning our first program, subtitled 'The Legal and Ethical Aspects of Medical Practice', we decided that the opening talk would be an 'Introduction to Medical Ethics'. Professor Richard Larkins, then Professor of Medicine at the Royal Melbourne Hospital, agreed to give the talk. I recall at the time being glad that I was not being asked to give this talk as my knowledge of the principles of medical ethics at that time was close to zero! I learned a large amount from Richard's excellent talk. Other topics covered in the course included medico-legal examinations and reports, medical certificates, drugs and poisons legislation, medical negligence, consent and informed decision making, the role of the Medical Board, ownership of medical records, complaint handling and certification of death. Through Vernon Plueckhahn's drive, all speakers responded to his request that their talk be made available in advance in printed form and each attendee thus received a complete folder of all the papers presented.

The first course was well attended but not by the young doctors we had hoped for. Despite our entreaties, no hospital took the initiative of releasing registrars to attend. The majority of the audience of around forty-five people were more senior doctors who had administrative responsibility at their hospitals for many of the subjects covered. Encouraged by this experience we ran the course again the following year, this time over just one and half days. We added extra themes including 'entering practice and practice management' and 'good communication skills'.

Our first book on medical practice, ethics and law

The organising committee then took stock of what we had been aiming for and what had been achieved. We decided that to continue the course each year was too labour intensive, especially as our initial target audience was not being reached. Vernon Plueckhahn suggested that as we now had a superb resource of many excellent papers, we should consider turning these into a text book and this is what was done. Once again, it was primarily Vernon Plueckhahn who took the lead in the editing, re-writing and new writing that was needed, with some assistance from Stephen Cordner and me. The book, entitled *'Law and Ethics in Medicine for Doctors in Victoria'* needed a publisher. Again, it was Vernon Plueckhahn who provided the solution by organising to self-publish it. Ian McVey undertook to raise the money to have sufficient copies printed so that every doctor in Victoria could receive a free copy and the Medical Board agreed to provide the addresses of those doctors. I was listed as one of the three editors. As this was a book partly about medical ethics, my 'career' as an untrained ethicist had probably begun.

It was soon to get a big push along. I had presented a paper on the Victorian Professional Practice Program to the inaugural conference of state and territory medical Boards, arranged by the NSW Medical Board in Sydney in late 1991, so our interstate colleagues were aware of this work. With the publication of our book in 1994, considerable interest was expressed in expanding the book to cover all Australian jurisdictions. This coincided with an unexpected change in my career direction such that I felt that I needed time out to decide what I should do next. I was entitled to six months long service leave from St Vincent's Hospital so I discussed with Vernon Plueckhahn and Stephen Cordner that I might take this leave and use it to expand our book to cover all the Australian states and territories. They readily accepted the idea. In 1996 I took long service leave and embarked on this project.

Vernon and Stephen remained deeply involved, editing and improving each chapter after I had revised the old or drafted most of the new ones. Our 1994 Victorian book had twelve chapters, most needing work to make them relevant nationally. Our new book had twenty-five chapters so there was plenty of research and writing to be done. The new chapters covered topics including the ethical and legal responsibilities of medical students, doctors' health, sexual misconduct, research in clinical practice, inter-professional relationships, maintenance of professional competence and the Australian health care system. It was during these six months that my in-depth exploration and self-teaching in medical ethics and medical law really took place. We were assisted in writing the book by many medical, legal, and regulatory colleagues around the nation who acted as content experts by critically reviewing the material that I had compiled for the revised and the new chapters. This was of vital importance to ensure accuracy and relevance.

We chose as the title for this edition *Ethics, Law and Medical Practice* and were able to enlist Allen and Unwin in Sydney as our publisher. The book was published in 1997. This was Allen and Unwin's first foray into medical textbooks and, although their editor was an enormous help to us, the quality and price of the book was very satisfactory, and the reviews, apart from one, were very positive, sales were slow. The only negative review came from a legal journal. We then realised that our title had failed to make it clear that the book was directed at doctors and not at lawyers. We may have aggravated this misjudgement by having Australia's best-known lawyer write a very generous foreword. Perhaps three non-lawyers writing about the law may have irked the legal reviewer. With regard to the slow sales, we were inclined to think that the publisher may not have had sufficient experience in marketing to doctors and medical students. Eventually the full print of 4,500 copies was sold. For several reasons it was to be another thirteen years before we published a new edition. When that finally happened, our new publisher suggested a much better title for the book.

I was now the first author of a textbook that, while not a text book of medical ethics, had a lot of ethical content. I was stumbling towards having a name as a medical ethicist even though I had not intended this. As confirmation of this lack of intent, I never joined and never attended any meetings of the Australian Bioethics Association* at any point in my career. I was not enamoured of the appearance on the Australian scene of medical ethicists and bioethicists and took a dim view (privately held) of some of them. I preferred to see myself as a clinician who was happy to engage in discussion and writing about issues surrounding professional conduct and misconduct and their intersection with ethical responsibilities. I did not feel capable of debating ethical theory and principles with all its associated jargon and terminology.

* The Australian Bioethics Association is now subsumed into the Australasian Association of Bioethics and Health Law.

The emergence of the field of bioethics

It was during the 1980s that the new academic field of bioethics emerged, with practitioners focussed in the first instance on ethical issues surrounding advances in biotechnology, especially in vitro fertilisation. Initially biotechnology was their sole focus. But it was not long before some of the participants saw that there was a vacuum in the more general field of medical ethics and were very willing to make pronouncements on any and every topic. At the time, in our medical schools and in post-graduate medical education, there was little or no focus on teaching medical ethics to medical students and young doctors; indeed, it was almost as if medical ethics as a subject or field of study was unimportant or non-existent. I also felt that through the use of highly academic and technical language, this new class of academic, the bioethicist, was having the effect of excluding clinicians from any role in public debate.

In Australia, an early development in bioethics was the establishment in 1980 of the Centre for Human Bioethics at Monash University, based in the Faculty of Arts, led by Professor Peter Singer and Dr Helga Kuhse. It was one of the first such centres in the world.[†] Peter Singer was adept at making provocative pronouncements and obtaining media attention, so soon the Centre and its work became well known. Singer played a key role in establishing the International Association of Bioethics in 1991, and its journal *Bioethics*. With Helga Kuhse, he founded the journal, *Monash Bioethics Review*, in 1982.

† The now well-known Hastings Centre in the USA and the Kennedy Centre, also in the USA, were established a little earlier, in 1969 and 1971 respectively.

Reflecting how new this field is, the Australian Bioethics Association held its first annual conference in 1991, the *American Journal of Bioethics* was only founded in 2001 and the New Zealand-based *Journal of Bioethical Inquiry* was founded in 2004.

In Sydney, the St James Ethics Centre (now in 2017 known simply as The Ethics Centre) was established in around 1990. Although having no credentials in clinical medicine and having as its goals working 'with individuals and families, organisations and industries, militaries and governments, to help people embed ethics at the centre of their choices and actions', the Centre's executive director was not averse to responding to the media's request for comment on what were essentially clinical or medical matters.

A small number of members of the medical profession around Australia now sought formal training in medical ethics and bioethics, and ethics centres gradually appeared in Australia, based generally in university faculties of medicine or in major teaching hospitals. The doctors and co-workers in these centres then played an active role in public debate and educational exchanges on ethical issues, relating not only to biotechnology but also broader medical practice. One of the first such centres was the Centre for Values, Ethics and Law in Medicine, based at the University of Sydney, led by highly regarded surgeon, Professor Miles Little, and established in 1995. The Plunkett Centre for Ethics, based at St Vincent's Public Hospital in Sydney preceded the University of Sydney Centre by three years. While the Plunkett centre has also been a very strong contributor to national debates, here I am focussing for the moment on medically-led centres.

By then there was also a solid cadre of faculty staff to teach medical ethics to medical students in all of Australia's medical schools. Mostly such teaching was provided in isolation from clinical teaching and one might wonder how much importance medical students, focussed on their learning for examinations, attached to such teaching. This seems to me to be another reason to seek to make all doctors comfortable with talking about ethical issues at the bedside.*

I have frequently observed that some doctors who sought training in medical ethics and then applied that new knowledge in dialogue with their medical colleagues were inclined to see their role as telling doctors 'what' to think rather than 'how' to think about any ethical issue, an approach that did not endear them to me. It contrasted quite markedly in my mind with the approach typically taken by a person trained in philosophy, and with an interest in medical ethics, who would see the need and indeed value in assisting any doctor to think their way through an issue. The problem that some medically qualified ethicists create for themselves in this way may be caused by their new self-image as a specialist in ethics and hence expected to have 'the' answers (as would a medical specialist giving clinical advice to a general practitioner). If they wished, such doctors could intimidate the recipients of their wisdom

* See two publications in the *Medical Journal of Australia* in 2001 which discuss how medical ethics teaching might best be provided to medical students: 'An ethics core curriculum for Australasian medical schools A Working Group, on behalf of the Association of Teachers of Ethics and Law in Australian and New Zealand Medical Schools (ATEAM)', *Medical Journal of Australia*, 2001, 175: 205–10 and 'Professional development and ethics for today's and tomorrow's doctors', *Medical Journal of Australia*, 2001, 175: 183–4.

by couching any advice in ethical jargon, thereby further emphasising the absence of educational dialogue.

An important milestone for Australia was the publication of a comprehensive text book of medical ethics for Australia by Dr Ian Kerridge and colleagues in 1998 with the title *Ethics and Law for the Health Professions*. Now in its fourth edition (2013), it is has gone from strength to strength, and has become the most important reference and educational source available for the medical and other health professions. Professor Kerridge now heads the Centre for Values, Ethics and Law in Medicine at the University of Sydney.

Chapter 4

MORE MEDICAL
BOARD EXPERIENCE

The appointment of non-medical members

My work on the Medical Board remained challenging and enjoyable throughout the 1980s and early 1990s. Many of the same members remained on the Board and the Board had a good sense of purpose and of camaraderie. We had had some success in requesting amendments to the legislation although we still had no control over staff selection or how the money that came in from the registration process was spent. Amendments to the Act passed in 1991 enlarged the Board membership to eleven people, providing for the appointment of a legally qualified member and a community member. The incoming Health Minister, Mrs Marie Tehan, appointed Mr John Stewart to the former position and Air Commodore David Smythe to the latter. Again demonstrating the various ways by which board members are appointed, both could trace their appointments to having served on other committees alongside Mrs Tehan. Both soon became effective contributors to the work of the Board.

From my work on the national edition of our text book, by then I had more knowledge about the professional difficulties doctors could get themselves into and more confidence about that knowledge. The initiative of the NSW Medical Board, led by Dr John Horvath, of the establishment of a biennial combined conference of all the Australian medical boards, first held in 1991, was stimulating all the boards to seek to improve their performance. Prior to this combined conference there was virtually no contact between medical board members from the other states. The board presidents did meet once or twice a year through the pathway of the Australian Medical Council and its Uniformity Committee (see Chapter 8).

An additional benefit that came from the first combined conference in Sydney was that the invited keynote speaker was the President of the US Federation of State Medical Boards, Dr Barbara Schneidman, whose visit was funded by the NSW Medical Board. Dr Schneidman gave a talk on doctors who are impaired (i.e. unwell and possibly not capable of practising safely). My only recall of her talk was her mention that, in the USA at that time, many state medical boards were dealing with allegations of sexual misconduct as a possible health or impairment issue in the doctor who was the subject of the allegations. This seemed to me to be fraught with risk as it overlooked the need first to protect the community. More relevantly, Dr Schneidman made us aware that Australian medical board members would be very welcome to attend the annual meeting of the US Federation as observers; indeed, John Horvath had already done so. I took the opportunity to make a self-funded trip in early 1994 and from that experience returned with a different view as to how doctors' health problems might be better handled.

As the Board had been asking government to appoint non-medical members for several years, the two new members were made very welcome and both were quickly able to make contributions at Board meetings. The modus operandi of the meetings was that each agenda item was allocated to a Board member ahead of the meeting and that member was expected to lead the discussion of the subject (these items were mostly new complaints). If a complaint related to a surgical matter, then a surgeon would lead the discussion. Non-medical members tended to be allocated complaints with little need for clinical knowledge, such as allegations of tardiness in providing medical reports, breaches of the dangerous drugs legislation and the like, and every effort was made to involve them fully in Board affairs. John Stewart frequently sat on Section 17 disciplinary inquiries where his legal expertise was put to good use, as was his talent for writing the Board's 'reasons for decision' document that was required after each inquiry.

It is difficult to measure the impact, internal or external, of having non-medical members on the Medical Board. One informal measure that I found very reassuring were the comments that virtually every new community or legal member made within a few months of joining. Most spoke in terms of joining the Board with the apprehension that the medical members would be 'soft' on doctors and yet what they observed was the opposite; i.e. they thought that we were too hard on those doctors about whom complaints had been lodged.

The arrival of the Health Services Commissioner

Another change that the Medical Board had to accommodate was the establishment in Victoria of the Office of the Health Service Commissioner in 1988 under the *Health Services (Conciliation and Review) Act 1987*. This was a first in Australia* and was welcomed by the Medical Board, especially for the reasons explained earlier that dissatisfied patients frequently were unsure where they should take their complaints in the first instance. Despite this welcome, there was a difficult initial period in establishing relationships between the Medical Board and the inaugural Health Services Commissioner, Dr Ian Siggins.

The practical stumbling block was that the legislation called for all complaints about registered medical practitioners to be 'shared' between the two agencies. This was achieved through the exchange of written complaints on their arrival (before any preliminary investigation) and then the Board President meeting with the Commissioner to agree which agency should handle the matter. This discussion hinged on whether the complaint was a matter suitable for conciliation or whether it raised issues of misconduct on the part of the doctor. Both the Board President and the Commissioner took seriously their responsibility to protect the public interest. However, the Board could not fail to notice that the Commissioner held a PhD but had no experience or training in any of the health professions, which, coupled with the other tensions,

---

* In NSW, a central health complaints office sited within the Health Department preceded the Victorian Commissioner but NSW did not establish its Health Care Complaints Commission until 1993.

meant that the Board struggled initially to have confidence in the office. Eventually relations improved and a de facto situation was agreed that the Board should take on those complaints which prima facie raised issues of public protection. In NSW, when a similar office was established in 1993, the legislation wisely provided a simple solution to this 'turf war' by stipulating that a complaint was to be handled by the agency that took the more serious view of it. Disagreements between the two agencies in Victoria were not just about personalities. Early in the time of the Commissioner who replaced Dr Siggins, I was deeply disturbed that the new appointee, a lawyer, was determined to hold on to a complaint of sexual misconduct and seek to conciliate it, without giving due regard to the need to protect future patients.

Taking on the Deputy Presidency

In 1991, Harry Garlick became unwell and sadly stepped down from membership of the Board. He was given a generous farewell dinner arranged by the Minister and the Health Department, an honour that he richly deserved. He had been a driving force for change and improvement in how the Board did its work. In deciding his replacement as Deputy President, the Minister sought the advice of the Board President, Bernard Neal, who then canvassed his fellow board members individually. The outcome was that I was appointed Deputy President. The fact that my name had gone forward after consultation with fellow members gave me confidence in accepting the role. I admired Bernard

Neal's chairmanship and was very happy to support him fully as his deputy. Unfortunately, I let him down on one occasion. I excuse my conduct by claiming that I was only following his example!

What happened was related to the link between the Medical Board and the Australian Medical Council (AMC). The AMC, established in 1985,* was in a way a child of the state and territory medical boards whose presidents constituted the majority of the Council's membership up until 2010. The key functions of the AMC at the outset were twofold; on behalf of the medical boards, to conduct examinations to assess the suitability of overseas trained doctors for registration by any state or territory medical board, and to accredit Australia's medical schools in order that their graduates were acceptable for registration. The AMC was funded in part through examination fees, in part by the Federal government, and in part by a levy on each medical board. It was the last of these sources of funding that led to my dilemma.

The inaugural president of the AMC was Dr Peter Livingstone, President of the Queensland Medical Board and the second was Dr Bernard Amos, President of the NSW Medical Board. In 1988, Dr Bernard Neal was elected President and served in this role until 1992. As President he chose to not share any of the deliberations of the AMC with his Victorian Medical Board colleagues. This approach came back to bite him when he took three months leave from the Medical Board in 1992, leaving me as Acting President.

---

* The Australian Medical Council's role, structure and history is described in *Assuring Medical Standards; The Australian Medical Council 1985–2010*, (ed.) Geffen, L. ISBN 978-1-875440-72-6.

While he was absent, we received our annual invoice from the AMC informing us what our contribution to the running costs of the AMC were to be and asking for payment. The amount asked was considerably more than in the previous year. This should not have been of great concern as the money came from consolidated revenue and not from the Medical Board which still had no money of its own. However, the letter hit some nerves that were raw, partly because the Board had no money and yet the AMC, now chaired by our own Board's President, could raise money simply by asking for it, and partly because Board members were irritated at being denied information about the workings of the AMC. Using Dr Neal's own chairmanship techniques, I let every Board member express their thoughts about the AMC's request for money. Having let the debate run, I was duty bound to accept a firm recommendation that the Victorian Board was unhappy with the steep increase in its contribution and that we request that the AMC revisit its budget and examine where savings might be made. An appropriate letter was sent to the AMC over my signature. Although I was aware that this approach was likely to upset and embarrass Dr Neal, deep down I was in favour of it. I had filled in for him at one AMC meeting and had realised that virtually all that was discussed could be freely shared with Victorian Board members. In due course Dr Neal returned from leave, discovered what had been done, and made it very clear at the first meeting of the Board that he was indeed angry and embarrassed. We survived that experience, and to his credit, the Executive Officer of the AMC revised his budget and sent us an invoice for a much smaller contribution.

Later, I too served on the AMC and I made sure that after every Council meeting, I briefed my fellow Board members in Victoria and answered any questions.

The second national conference of medical boards

In 1993, the Victorian Medical Board convened the second national conference of state and territory medical boards, following on the successful NSW conference. Dr Neal must have been losing his enthusiasm for his role as he declined to take part in planning the conference and asked me to chair the program committee. Like our NSW counterpart, we too were keen to invite a significant international speaker. Rather than turning again to the USA, we sent a letter of invitation to the President of the General Medical Council (GMC) of the UK, which was graciously accepted. Our lack of knowledge of the UK regulatory scene became apparent when he and his wife flew to Melbourne. The President, a knight of the realm and a physician, was elderly, not physically well and soon to complete his term of office. He was a very pleasant man but in the one talk he gave, which was about the very beginnings in the UK of a process now known as revalidation,* it seemed to me that he had not been deeply involved in its development. From what I was to learn later, we would have been wiser to invite the Registrar of the GMC who could have spoken with much

_____

* The proposed new UK process of revalidation, which translates as a means of documenting that any doctor is keeping his or her knowledge and skills up-to-date, was put to the 1993 Victorian conference as something that was imminent. Revalidation was finally put in place in the UK in 2012. See: Revalidation – what is the problem and what are the possible solutions? Breen, K J, *Medical Journal of Australia*, vol. 200, 2014, pp. 153–6.

more knowledge and authority on this and other topics and would have been a more energetic participant in conference discussions.

Much later, and with many events that subsequently transpired in the UK, I formed the view that in 1993, the GMC had been in the doldrums. Its handling of complaints was antiquated and weighted heavily in the favour of doctors. It had poor processes for handling misconduct that fell short of very serious. It was well behind the regulatory changes that were proceeding in Canada, USA and Australia. It relied too heavily on the UK National Health Service processes for handling complaints and for assessing possibly impaired doctors. And it probably suffered from the inbuilt class system that led most of the UK patient population not to challenge the decisions of doctors or of the GMC. There were to be many wake-up calls including events known now as Bristol,[†] Alder Hey[‡] and the Shipman

[†] The deaths of 29 babies undergoing heart surgery at the Bristol Royal Infirmary in the late 1980s and early 1990s led to a major inquiry in 1998 that resulted in extensive recommendations for reform in the NHS. As reported in the Guardian, the inquiry 'lifted the lid on an 'old boy's' culture among doctors; patients being left in the dark about their treatment; a lax approach to clinical safety; low priority given to children's services; secrecy about doctor's performance, and a lack of external monitoring of NHS performance'. See https://www.theguardian.com/society/2002/jan/17/5 . See also the full report http://webarchive.nationalarchives.gov.uk/20090811143822/http://www.bristol-inquiry.org.uk/final_report/the_report.pdf. The inquiry became an examination not only of the Bristol hospital but also of the NHS and the regulation of the medical profession in the UK.

[‡] The Alder Hey Children's Hospital scandal and subsequent inquiry was about the unauthorised retention of body parts during 1988 to 1995. See https://en.wikipedia.org/wiki/Alder_Hey_organs_scandal. The Alder Hey scandal later had an im-

case.* None of these scandals directly involved the GMC at their outset but the events and the inquiries that followed shook the British medical establishment, which very much included the GMC, forcing the Council to reform many of its processes.

The only thing that the GMC was doing well in the 1990s was addressing instances of research misconduct by doctors and even that responsibility was forced upon it. During the 1990s, I was a regular reader of the *British Medical Journal* (which now calls itself the *BMJ*) and still am today. The journal included a weekly news column which covered, among many items, the outcome of GMC disciplinary hearings. I was impressed and puzzled as to how many hearings involved doctors charged with defrauding drug companies by deceptive conduct of clinical trials. While there was mounting concern in other countries over such conduct, the GMC was the only medical board prosecuting doctors. It was to be years before I stumbled across the explanation for this difference.† The Association of the British Pharmaceutical Industry had hired a talented investigator. When his findings in many cases were

---

pact in Australia as many hospitals here stored body parts for teaching purposes. In Australia at that time, the consent of family was not deemed necessary, so these parts had been retained legally. However, community attitudes had changed and reform was necessary. Chapter 9 describes the impact of the Alder Hey affair in Australia.

* Dr Harold Shipman was found guilty of murdering fifteen patients and it was later estimated that he may have deliberately killed up to 250 patients. The Shipman Inquiry recommended changes to the structure of the General Medical Council. See https://en.wikipedia.org/wiki/Harold_Shipman.

† Wells, F, 'Historical aspects of research misconduct: Europe', in *Fraud and Misconduct in Biomedical Research*, Wells, F and Farthing, M (eds.), 4th edn., Royal Society of Medicine Press, London, 2008.

submitted to the GMC, it was forced to take action.

Regulatory change was indeed afoot in Australia. The Cain/Kirner ALP government in Victoria had established a working party in 1991 to advise the government on a new *Medical Practice Act*. The Medical Board was represented on the working party by Dr Neal. I gained an insight into the difficulties Dr Neal faced in putting across to the working party the desired improvements that the current Medical Board was hoping for when I filled in for him for a single meeting one evening. The meeting was chaired eccentrically by the then Health Services Commissioner who emphasised his approach to chairmanship by suddenly announcing at around 7.30 pm that he was off to the theatre and the rest of us should simply carry on in his absence! I also observed that the committee appeared heavily biased in favour of lawyers associated with the Health Issues Centre[‡] and that there seemed to be a strong determination to take the regulation of doctors out of the hands of the medical profession. I went home disillusioned and depressed.

Luckily, help was at hand in the form of a state election in 1992, where Joan Kirner's ALP was replaced by Jeff Kennett's Liberals and Mrs Marie Tehan became Minister for Health. I do not recall what process Mrs Tehan used to develop the 1994 *Medical Practice Act* but I do recall that she accepted virtually all the recommendations made by the Medical Board. As discussed in a subsequent chapter, these included a much more humane and personalised approach to dealing with unwell and impaired doctors.

---

‡ The Health Issues Centre, established in 1983, is the key health consumer advocacy agency in Victoria. In its early days, I sensed that it was strongly linked to the left side of Victorian politics.

Chapter 5

The 1994 Medical Practice Act

Big changes arrive

The Victorian *Medical Practice Act* of 1994 brought many changes. Under the new Act, the Board, now renamed the Medical Practitioners Board of Victoria, became fully independent from the Health Department. This meant that new premises had to be found, staff had to be hired and the Board had to fund its operations through the receipt of doctors' registration fees. The new Act altered the manner in which impaired doctors were handled and made changes to the way in which complaints were dealt with and disciplinary hearings were conducted. Section 17 inquiries under the previous Act became 'formal hearings' under the new Act and were now to be open to the public. The number of Board members was increased by one, a second community member, bringing the membership to twelve.

The new Act took effect from July 1994 and coincided with the date at which several three-year Board memberships were due for reappointment. Two long-serving members, the President, Bernard Neal, and surgeon, John Clarebrough, chose not to seek reappointment and were farewelled with fine dinners. I was invited by Health Minister Tehan to take over as President, a task that I was willing to accept. The timing was fortunate in one key aspect. For the previous eighteen months, I had been deeply involved in a major review and overhaul as to how patient care was to be delivered in a new building at St. Vincent's Hospital due to open in 1995. The new building was to house all clinical services apart from the outpatient clinics, the rehabilitation block and mental health services.

My involvement in the project at St Vincent's was to a large degree serendipitous. At the time, I was one of two medical members of the staff at St Vincent's on its inaugural Board of Directors. The more senior medical member had a fear of flying and declined an invitation to take part in a ten-day study tour of US hospitals. I was asked to replace him. The hospital CEO, Dr David Campbell, participated in the same tour. I found the tour very enlightening. Having previously worked in the USA, I was familiar with the strengths and weaknesses of American health care, so I was in a good position to discern new approaches to hospital work processes that might be valuable for the new St. Vincent's. I wrote a ten-page report of my experience and ideas and sent it to Dr Campbell. I was surprised when he phoned me a couple of days later praising my report and asking if he could add his name to it and submit it to the Board of Directors as the official report of the study tour. The report became the basis for what was eventually called the St Vincent's Patient Care Project,* a project that I co-directed.

The period 1992–6 were rewarding years and also very difficult years, professionally and personally, for me.

* Campbell, D H and Breen, K J, Patient Care Model Project: St Vincent's Hospital, Melbourne, *Journal of the Australian Hospital Association*, 1994, 17, 57–66.

Towards the end of that period, I was possibly experiencing symptoms of burnout. These were also years of major changes at St Vincent's Hospital. For its first 100 years, St Vincent's was owned and conducted by the Catholic religious order of nuns, the Sisters of Charity. A Sister was appointed by the order to run the hospital, effectively serving in a role that the combined the responsibilities of a Board of Directors and a Chief Executive Officer. Recruits to the order had dropped enormously and at the start of the last decade of the twentieth century, the Sisters of Charity made the difficult decision to withdraw from directly running the hospital. Instead the hospital would become an incorporated entity with a Board of Directors which would appoint a CEO to take charge of the hospital. In 1991 this change took place and I found myself as one of two medical staff members on the new Board.

As part of the restructuring of the hospital that was associated with incorporation, I was appointed in 1992 to a half-time management position as Executive Chairman of the Division of Medicine. It took me four years to realise that I was not well-suited to this role but in the meanwhile I participated in a change program, including the Patient Care Model project described above, that had the effect of designing myself out of this job. In taking on the Executive Chairman role, I briefly continued in my role as Director of the Department of Gastroenterology but stepped down from that position when the Patient Care Model project began in 1993.

My service on the inaugural Board of Directors of St Vincent's only lasted twelve months. Shortly after I accepted the management position as Executive Chairman of the

Division of Medicine, I was invited to a meeting by the Chairman of the Board of Directors and the newly appointed CEO. The Chairman informed me that the new CEO was uncomfortable that a staff member who reported to him (i.e. yours truly) was serving on the Board to which he reported. It was put to me that I should resign from the Board. Instead of seeking time to think this decision through or get advice, I agreed. Soon after, I found that my colleague, Executive Director of the Division of Surgery, the late Dr John Doyle, was made of sterner stuff and had declined the invitation to resign. I was probably better off to be free of this additional duty. My only regret was that I missed a 'ringside seat' to some turbulent years.

Not only was I too busy for my own good at this time which also covered my term as Deputy President of the Medical Board and my acceptance of the Presidency of the Medical Practitioners Board in July 1994, but I was also facing personal stresses. My youngest child, a son aged 18, had suddenly become critically ill in early 1993 and required three major operations, the first life-saving, during the next twelve months. A year or so later my marriage of 24 years faltered. There was no lack of warning signs that my life was out of control. During this period, I once found myself booked for three different meetings scheduled at the exactly the same time, and on another occasion I missed an international flight by 24 hours. I heeded the warnings eventually and took six months long service leave at the start of 1996. I never returned to a fulltime hospital appointment nor to a hospital management position. I am sure that my wish to avoid confrontation made me unsuitable for a hospital management role that often involved saying no to the quite reasonable requests of colleagues for increased resources.

However, my role in the Patient Care Model Project had some timely benefits. Through engagement in this project, I became aware if expertise was needed in a particular area, then provided one had the money, expertise could be hired short-term or long-term. The project had involved considerable effort in communicating with hospital staff and I had learnt about the value of expertise in communication and public relations. I sensed that this was going to be important for the new Medical Practitioners Board because, after over 100 years of existence, the Board was finally to be exposed to media scrutiny.

How the new Medical Practitioners Board might be improved

In accepting the appointment as Board president, I already had several ideas as to how the Board might improve its work. I was happy that the Board's formal hearings were to be open to the media as I felt that the Board needed to be more visible to the public and the profession. I had formed ideas as to how the Board might be able to do more for impaired doctors and to better handle sexual misconduct cases. While the new Board contained a couple of medical members who held quite conservative traditional views about the role of the Board, I was very happy with the membership that I had been given and felt optimistic about the future.

From the outset we were treated very badly by the Health Department and the Kennett government in one important respect. Board members expected that in our first year of operation, we would collect and use the annual renewal of registration fees, now to be paid in October, to finance our operations. However, to our dismay, we were told that such fees were to be apportioned retrospectively to pay for the previous year's expenses incurred by the Health Department. In my view, this was a truly amazing stunt performed by the government solely for the purpose of stealing $1.5 million from the unsuspecting medical profession. We sought behind the scenes to involve the Victorian AMA to lobby on our behalf, but at that time, Kennett's powers were at their height and the AMA was reluctant to fight a public battle. The new Board was thus coerced into borrowing $1.5 million at 9% interest rate to be paid off over four years. This meant that in the new Board's first year of operating we had to have a striking increase in annual renewal of registration fees. Naturally, this was not well received by the doctors of Victoria.

In my few dealings with Health Minister, Marie Tehan, I found her manner a little prickly. While Bernard Neal was still President, she gave us a community Board member whom I presumed she must have known personally. It seemed that he felt he had been given a personal mandate from the Minister to take charge of the transition processes that were required for the new *Medical Practice Act*. He fell out with his colleagues and resigned from the Board, not long before the new Medical Practitioners Board was formed. A few months later, the new Board held an official opening of its premises in South Melbourne at which Minister Marie Tehan spoke. We invited a large number of people but after consulting with Board colleagues, it was felt that if we sent an invitation to the member who had recently resigned we might be seen to be 'rubbing salt into a wound', so he was not invited. Mrs Tehan noticed his absence and wrote me an unpleasant letter without ever inquiring as to why he had not been invited, why he had resigned, or the circumstances surrounding his resignation.

On the other hand, in defence of Mrs Tehan, the Board benefited enormously from her appointment of Mr John Stewart as our first legally qualified Board member (he was also a qualified accountant). John was a delightful man, thoughtful, helpful and knowledgeable, and a great team person. He was loved and respected by all. His premature death from cancer in 2000 was a tragic loss. Mrs Tehan attended his funeral and was very pleasant when we met there. Later she also gave us an excellent community member, Miss Rae Anstee, who like John Stewart was a tower of strength on the Board.

In the early work on a new Act undertaken by a committee appointed by the previous ALP government, the Medical Board had been threatened with losing the power to hold disciplinary hearings into allegations of serious misconduct. The idea was that this power would be given to an independent tribunal. Under the *Medical Practice Act* 1994, this power remained with the Medical Practitioners Board. I am aware of, and readily appreciate, the argument that the medical board should not be investigator, prosecutor and judge of misconduct allegations. (This argument eventually held sway when another Act – the *Health Professions Registration Act* – came into operation in 2007.) However, at the time, I argued against this change for pragmatic reasons which included my belief that this broader role made for a greater sense of responsibility among Board members, increased their capacity to see the 'big picture', and increased their job satisfaction. I was concerned that an independent tribunal led by a lawyer or judge might not be able to readily recruit medical members of high standing to serve on its panels.

Inquiries into more serious allegations of misconduct were now called 'formal hearings' for which the Board was obliged to form a panel of a minimum of three members, one to be legally qualified, one to be a community member and at least one a medical practitioner. In practice panels were usually composed of four people, two being medical practitioners. Formal hearings panels were still to be chaired by a medically qualified Board member and this task was usually allocated to the President or Deputy President. The presence of a legally qualified member of a panel, usually John Stewart, was of great assistance, especially when a barrister appearing for a doctor tried to bluff the panel with complex legal argument. The new Act made clear that formal hearings were to be open to the public (meaning the media). The new Act also shifted the site of appeals against Board disciplinary decisions from the Victorian Supreme Court to the Victorian Civil and Administrative Tribunal (VCAT), and made the appeal a complete re-hearing, a change that initially caused the Medical Practitioners Board some alarm.

Appeals against decisions of the Board

The new Board may have been oversensitive to the outcome of appeals because of the result of an appeal against the last decision made by the old Medical Board. Not long before we transitioned to the new *Medical Practice Act*, an appeal by a doctor to the Supreme Court demonstrated how far apart the legal and medical profession can be. The doctor, recently divorced, had had a sexual relationship with a depressed and vulnerable female patient and had not denied the relationship. The Medical Board found the doctor guilty of serious professional misconduct and suspended his registration for six months. The judge who heard the appeal was about to retire. He found in the doctor's favour in that he reduced the penalty to a reprimand. In my view, this was a terrible decision and was tantamount to saying that it is acceptable for doctors to use their examination room as a place to find people to date. Incidentally, it turned out to be the only Board disciplinary decision that I was involved in during my 19 years of service that was altered or overturned on appeal.

Thus, with this recent experience in mind, the Board was anxious as to how VCAT would handle its first hearings of appeals from decisions of the Medical Practitioners Board. For the first few appeals, VCAT chose to appoint a single legal member to hear the appeals. To us this seemed extremely unbalanced when one considered that cases originally had been decided by a three or more person panel of the Board containing experienced doctors and a legal member. It was not possible as a member or head of a statutory body like the Medical Practitioners Board to approach VCAT directly to raise our concerns and neither was it acceptable or wise to use the media to draw attention to such concerns. We had to use informal channels of communication to express these concerns which we did via a number of paths. There was never any public acknowledgement but soon afterwards VCAT started conducting their hearings using an additional medically qualified member. This was a step in the right direction although VCAT chose a relatively junior psychiatrist who was already a member of VCAT for other reasons, a person with no experience of professional misconduct matters. Under the law in place currently, VCAT is now the primary tribunal hearing allegations of serious misconduct and its panels routinely are made up of a lawyer and two medical practitioners.

On almost every occasion that the subject of appeals against medical board or medical tribunal disciplinary decisions is open to review and public comment, one finds otherwise well-informed people, including some lawyers, arguing that just as the doctor concerned has a right of appeal, so also should the patient who lodged the complaint. This is argued so often that eventually a parliament will kow-tow even though in my view this is a totally inappropriate means for any unhappy patient gaining redress. The key principle to remember here is that, at the medical board or medical tribunal hearing, the only person with anything to lose (by way of registration and/or reputation and livelihood) is the doctor. The complainant has no stake in the hearing other than through being prepared to give evidence that the doctor may have acted unprofessionally. The complainant faces no bill for legal representation and at most might be inconvenienced by aggressive cross-examination. To suggest that this person is entitled to appeal should the doctor be exonerated of unprofessional conduct is to completely misunderstand the purpose of disciplinary proceedings. Should there exist potentially valid reasons for a complainant to remain dissatisfied or injured by the doctors' conduct, the civil courts are where this person should head.

The new Board and its work

The new Board in 1994 was different from the old in many ways. We now had control over our budget and control over whom we employed. Prior to this time, the Board was totally dependent on the Department of Health for staff who were allocated to us and we had gone through very difficult times with progressive staff cuts. We took with us our long serving public servant, Board Registrar Mr John Smith, into this new independent world. John was an extremely hard-working person who was very familiar with the work of the Board and we felt that with all the challenges ahead we needed his experience. He courageously forwent the benefits of working in the public service and joined the staff in South Melbourne. He was ably supported by Ms Rose Siecris, an accountant who was recruited to establish our accounting, payroll, and registration renewal processes, and to oversee meeting our information technology needs.

One thing that did not change with the new *Medical Practice Act* was the amount of work undertaken by Board members on an honorary basis. Members were paid only for attending at Board meetings, disciplinary hearings and subcommittee meetings. The payment, regulated by government, was minimal. Preparation for Board meetings, which involved reading a large folder of papers every two weeks, and tasks such as writing reasons for decisions of formal hearings, were unpaid. The chair of the Health Committee, who was required to undertake a lot of work outside of Board meetings, did this on an honorary basis. As President, I was in the Board's office two or three times a week outside the days of Board meetings for which there was no remuneration. Until 1996, I was still a full-time employee of St Vincent's Hospital so in a way the hospital was subsidising the work of the Board. I understand that the new President from the year 2000 was paid an honorarium for such duties.

We had legislated authority to work in subcommittees and we established several, including a health committee, a publications committee, a registration committee and a finance and audit committee. John Stewart chaired the finance and audit committee, a task he performed very efficiently. Dr Bryce Phillips was Deputy President and he chaired the registration committee. He also took on his share of chairing formal disciplinary hearings. I never sat with him as chair but I understood that his style was quite different from mine. Formal hearings varied in length, with most running about two or three days. The longest hearing I ever chaired ran for 41 days, while the most distressing hearing was an undefended case involving a male psychiatrist who had engaged in sexual misconduct with several young vulnerable female patients. As chair of any hearing panel, I used to write many of the 'reasons for decision' documents. This task was shared with lawyer member, John Stewart. These documents needed a lot of care as Board decisions were subject to appeal.

The Board also had a statutory committee, the Intern Accreditation Committee (IAC), which oversaw and accredited intern training posts in Victorian hospitals. A member of the Medical Board was required to chair this committee. Leading up to 1994, this position had been held by an experienced but now retired medical administrator. I felt that the intern training committee was 'coasting' under his leadership and I took the difficult decision to ask him to stand down in favour of a Board member with a fresh perspective and a track record in medical education. While he took this reasonably well, my working relationship with him was never the same. The new Board from 1994 had a system of rotation whereby each year, four of the now twelve members were to retire. This member was not reappointed a year or so later and the tension I had felt was no longer an issue. Board member, Dr Joanna Flynn, was appointed as the new chair of the IAC and did a very good job.

The importance of good public relations

Weighing heavily on my mind was how the Board was going to handle its relationship with the media. I was very fortunate that the Board approved the appointment of an outstanding public relations and communications adviser, Ms Nicole Newton, who (again serendipitously) I had met through the Patient Care Project at St Vincent's Hospital. Nicole was instrumental in much of the good work done in the following years. The new *Medical Practice Act* meant that formal disciplinary hearings (i.e. those devoted to more serious allegations of professional misconduct) now had to be open to the public. We debated as a Board how this should best occur. I felt that we needed to be as transparent as possible and that this meant we should announce open hearings in the daily newspapers, in the section devoted to the 'Law List'. There was opposition to such openness by some Board members and it was only Nicole Newton's eloquent advice to the Board as how any other approach would be seen very negatively by the media that won the day.

I have no doubt that the coverage which sometimes accompanies disciplinary hearings is very unpleasant for the medical practitioner involved but that is one of the prices to be paid for the right to self-regulation. Media coverage is unpredictable. I recall a formal hearing (possibly involving allegations of sexual misconduct, but I am now not sure) where interest from one media outlet was high but no coverage resulted. It turned out that, on the way to the Board premises, the journalist was redirected to a crime scene in the northern suburbs!

Another aspect of media coverage relates to the usual sequence of adversarial legal proceedings. On day one of any proceeding, the allegations are read out and an outline of the evidence against the doctor is provided. This information becomes the basis for the initial report in the media thereby creating a negative impression of the doctor. Subsequent evidence in favour of the doctor receives less or no attention, likewise a finding that the allegations are found to be not substantiated. Experienced journalist and past editor in chief of the Melbourne *Age*, Ranald Macdonald, described this unfairness accurately in 2017 when he wrote 'My mantra has always been that fairness and factual accuracy is Journalism 101. Tell me how you achieve balance when you rely on sources, tip offs and in covering a story which is still unfolding – and how is it possible to get daily 'balance' in reporting, for example, court cases? There, the prosecution makes absolutely clear at the outset that the Defendant is guilty – then later the defence puts its case and often casts compelling doubts on his/her guilt. Reporters give the dramatic first day 'lead' by outlining the crime, the prosecution's case and the 'perpetrator' – unless editors are ethically observant and strive for fairness, the drama of the accusation overwhelms what follows. Even when there is a not guilty verdict'.* Macdonald's remarks apply equally to medical tribunal hearings.

In my view, most media coverage in my time as President of the Board was even-handed, and for this again I need to acknowledge the behind the scenes work which Nicole Newton put into briefing journalists about the processes and the powers of the Medical Practitioners Board. I am annoyed at myself for having lost the reference as there was an interesting study reported from the UK several years ago which examined community attitudes to doctors who had been the subject of adverse publicity when appearing before the GMC. My recollection of the study was that the general public seemed to have quite short memories for such publicity and did not continue to be concerned about what they had heard or read.

The composition of the Medical Practitioners Board was very much in the hands of the Minister of the day. As President, I worked with three ministers, Mrs Marie Tehan, Mr Rob Knowles and, briefly, Mr John Thwaites. With Minister Tehan, you got the members she chose, while with Minister Knowles, there was consultation with the President. The Board had at times had a couple of members who seemed unsuited to their role and who struggled to contribute. Fortunately, there was a practice, which I was

*   http://johnmenadue.com/ranald-macdonald-abc-deal-comes-back-to-haunt-the-government-episode-two/.

happy to continue, of allocating agenda items at each Board meeting to a Board member who was expected to have researched the topic and who would lead the debate. This meant that I was able to allocate the more problematic issues to the best people. I also had control over who would chair disciplinary hearings, sit on hearing panels and serve on board committees so I could usually work my way around our few 'weak links'.

I had a great respect and liking for Health Minister Mr Rob Knowles. He was an open person, not given to political wheeling and dealing, and one who seemed to want to listen to the Board's views. He was supportive of the work of the Board and easy to work with. We had an effective working relationship although the number of times there needed to be contact was infrequent. His first Parliamentary Secretary for Health was Dr Dennis Napthine (introduced publicly one day by a fellow Board member as Dr 'Napthalene'). His next Parliamentary Secretary accepted an invitation to meet with the members of the Board. This proved to be somewhat disappointing as, in the allotted time, we learnt quite a lot about the Parliamentary Secretary but there was little time left for him to learn of the work of the Board and the problems the Board faced.

My contact with Health Minister John Thwaites was only over a short period of time. He was receptive to hearing my views on who my fellow Board members, whom I had consulted individually, felt were the two best qualified people to be considered for the Presidency of the Board when I stepped down in mid-2000. He also very generously allowed me to stay on the Board as an ordinary member for an additional six months until the end of 2000 in order that I could complete my three year term as President of the Australian Medical Council.

The transition from the old world to the new was overall uncontentious. Nevertheless, there were two members of the Board who had served in the old world and who felt the need to object to some of the changes. They led the objection to announcing formal hearings in the law list. They also sought to make their presence felt in another way. In separating from the Department of Health, the Board needed to have its own stationery and logo. We engaged a design firm to undertake this work and they came up with a very attractive, simple and clean logo and colour scheme. The design included a traditional symbol of medicine known as the image of Aesculapius, which is an image of a serpent wound around a staff. The Board meeting was tied up for thirty minutes as these two traditionalists argued that the image should have two serpents and not one!

For my own education, and because of the work involved in our textbook, I was a keen reader of the international literature on medical regulation, especially as mentioned, the news section of the *British Medical Journal*. I was a little surprised and perhaps disappointed that this interest seemed not to be shared by my fellow Board members. I determined that this might change. The Board accepted my advice that it would benefit from access to a medical library. I had already had the benefit of access to the library and librarian at the Victorian Institute of Forensic Medicine and through my contact with the Institute Director, Professor Stephen Cordner, the Institute agreed for a very small fee to act as the library for the Medical Board. The librarian extracted and photocopied the list of contents of several key journals and these were circulated each fortnight with the Board's agenda papers. If I or any Board member came across an article that appeared relevant to the work of the Board, a copy of that article would be circulated for the next meeting. I have no idea what impact this had on my fellow Board members and I don't think that my successor continued this service.

It has long been important for the Medical Board to have the confidence of the profession, especially its peak body, the Victorian Branch of the Australian Medical Association. Good fortune fell my way again as, at about the time I was appointed President of the Board, Dr Robyn Mason became CEO of AMA Victoria. I knew Robyn well as she had been a medical administrator at St Vincent's Hospital. We trusted each other and thus were able to discuss issues of mutual concern fully and frankly. This was very useful as, in formal situations, leaders of AMA Victoria may have to posture to an audience and thus it was crucial that AMA Victoria understood the Board's stance and reasoning on key issues. AMA Victoria was able to lobby the Health Minister on our behalf if needed.

Equally valuable to me was the fact that the incoming President of the Medical Defence Association of Victoria (MDAV) at about that time was orthopaedic surgeon, Mr Robert Dickens, whom I had known for many years. One of MDAV's tasks is to support doctors facing disciplinary action by the Board and in that role, there of course could be no contact over specific cases. However, it was in the interests of both agencies that we had a clear understanding of each other's positions on more general matters, and we were able to work very effectively with MDAV and the other indemnity providers.

Good fortune also favoured me with the two Health Services Commissioners with whom I worked between 1994 and 2000 when I served as Board President. The first was Acting Commissioner, Ms Vivienne McCutcheon, who filled the role for more than a year after ill-health unfortunately interrupted Ms Lisa Newby's term of office. Ms McCutcheon was followed by Ms Beth Wilson. Both were a pleasure to work with and fully understood and valued the public protection role of the Medical Practitioners Board. The discussions each fortnight about the latest complaints received, and how we could best address these, were amicable and always based on what was in the best interests of the community.

Under the new *Medical Practice Act*, the responsibilities of the Board and its staff had increased considerably. Staff numbers had also increased. Staff now had to handle the entire process of annual renewal of registration, the payroll, media relations, Board publications and the like. The Board decided that the registrar was badly overloaded and needed senior help. This was to be achieved through recruitment of a chief executive officer, leaving the registrar with the primary responsibility of managing the complaints section and disciplinary hearings, matters in which he was expert from many years of responsibility. The Board then made two additional decisions that may have been unwise. We decided that we should try to have the CEO in place ahead of a planned relocation from South Melbourne to Lonsdale Street in the city, a move that was imminent. We decided also to use a recruitment agency to search for our CEO.

Finding reasons to move on

I was disappointed with the quality of the applicants for the CEO position. But as we had signed up with the agency, the Board's five-member selection committee, which I chaired, decided to go ahead with the planned interviews of the short list that the agency had identified. In the lead up to this day, I had spoken with the head of the recruitment agency on a couple of occasions and had formed an impression that he had only one candidate in mind. None of the candidates had any experience in the regulation of health professionals or like experience. In hindsight we probably should have declined to make an appointment and readvertised but we did not. Instead we appointed the candidate who interviewed the best. He began in the position in mid-1999 just ahead of our relocation.

Soon after that, I authorised a document that he had written on my behalf, informing doctors of the move to Lonsdale Street, to be mailed without my close vetting and editing. This was my mistake. In announcing the new Board offices, he had used words to the effect of 'premises suitable for such a prestigious profession' or something along those lines. Many doctors read the letter and gained the impression that the Board was wasting money on luxury office space for itself. I received some angry letters from senior members of the medical profession and replied promptly and as apologetically as I could. After this bruising experience, I harboured doubts about whether I could fully trust the judgement of the CEO. However, I had been party to the appointment process and I had to live with it.

My inability to relate well with our CEO did help me to

make another important decision. In July 2000, I would have been President for two three-year terms and a member of the Board for nineteen years. While I may have had the energy and enthusiasm to seek a third three-year term as President, I was not fully confident of that. Also, I felt that if I stayed another three years, the two best candidates available to replace me may have moved on. Combining these thoughts with my uncomfortable relationship with the CEO eventually made my decision an easy one and I stepped down as President in July 2000 and left the Board at the end of the year.

Looking back, I think there was another reason why I had difficulty in working with the CEO, a reason that lay within me and not the CEO. I had been a very 'hands on' president, partly because I can't resist trying to perform any task to the best of my ability and partly because of the extent of the work involved in the transition in 1994 from a Board supported by the Department of Health to a fully independent Board. In a way, I had at times probably been both the Board President and its CEO. Having a new CEO meant that I was always likely to have trouble giving up that part of my role. I am sure that the CEO was happy to see me move on.

As mentioned above, I came to the position as President with the thought that the new Board might be able to do more for doctors who were unwell and possibly impaired and do better in handling allegations of sexual misconduct. Thanks to the energy and support of several members of the Board, we were able to make significant progress in both areas. As these two subjects are important in their own right, they are discussed later in separate chapters.

Chapter 6

HEALTH ISSUES OF DOCTORS

Dealing with the impaired doctor

With the advent of the new 1994 *Medical Practice Act*, the processes by which the Medical Board handled doctors who were unwell and possibly impaired were theoretically made less stressful. As mentioned earlier, the term 'impaired' refers to the inability of the doctor to practise safely and competently. This change to the legislation was made in response to representations from the Medical Board as the Board believed that this would result in doctors seeking help earlier in their illnesses. When notified of a possibly impaired doctor, the Board was now empowered to appoint one of its members to communicate with that doctor directly and in person, a much more humane approach than calling the unfortunate doctor to appear before the entire Board. Most of this work was done by our health subcommittee, chaired initially by psychiatrist, Dr Channa Wijesinghe, and later by physician, Dr John Court. The nominated Board member's task was to arrange for an independent report from an appropriate specialist who was asked to advise on the doctor's fitness to remain in practice and about any conditions that the Board might need to place on the doctor's registration that would ensure community safety. The independent report was provided to the doctor and to the Board member who would discuss the report and any recommendations with the doctor concerned. Almost universally, the unwell doctor was prepared to accept the recommendations of the independent specialist, in which case (subject to the approval of the health subcommittee) they became the Board's recommendations.

To give some flavour of the cases handled, the two common examples were doctors who had become addicted to narcotic drugs such as pethidine or to alcohol, and doctors with a serious mental illness such as recurrence of a psychosis, for example, schizophrenia or bipolar disorder. The Board and its health subcommittee took a firm attitude to drug addiction as past experience had taught the Board two key lessons. First, withdrawal from any drug was nigh on impossible if the doctor sought to keep working, so the Board had a policy of immediate suspension and directing the doctor to seek treatment. Second, relapse in the first twelve months was not unusual but this was not necessarily a sign of a bad prognosis. It seemed that some doctors needed such a relapse to drive home to them how serious was the problem they faced.

While some doctors are inclined to harshly judge colleagues who become severely stressed or depressed or who self-administer drugs of dependence, this is not fair or appropriate in my view. My view is heavily influenced by research published by American psychiatrist, Dr George Vaillant and colleagues in 1972.* They conducted a prospective 30-year study comparing 47 doctors with 79 socio-economically matched controls in professions other than medicine. Their findings indicated that doctors at risk of burnout, anxiety and depression, substance abuse and addiction, or marriage breakdown are often also doctors who take their caring role very seriously and exhibit greater empathy and altruism to patients than their more resilient colleagues. The research suggested that, for many of these doctors, unresolved emotional issues dating back to unhappy childhoods led them to seek to use the caring role in medicine to compensate for this loss. When I first read the paper of Vaillant, it did not cross my mind that the research findings might apply to my own situation; this insight came much later in my career.

The various stresses of medical practice seem to have increased during my life as a doctor. I suggest that some of the increased stress is linked to increased expectations of better educated patients together with increased regulation of doctors. I don't for one moment deplore most of these changes and mention them only to support my view that the practice of medicine has become more stressful. If you have any doubt about how stressful some events in medical practice might be then pause for a moment and ask yourself how you would feel if faced with an appearance in the Coroner's Court or at a medical tribunal hearing, or of being named in the media because a patient was suing you for negligence.

During my period as President of the Medical Practitioners Board, doctors who were severely psychotic often created

* Vaillant, G E, Sobowale, N C, 'McArthur C. Some psychologic vulnerabilities of physicians', N Eng J Med, 287, 1972: 372–5.

trouble for the Board, because with the illness came loss of insight into their situation. If the doctor was in a psychiatric hospital, the community was not at risk. But as many were under community treatment orders, the monitoring of the strict conditions placed on their registration became more difficult. Many were the times when the chair of our health committee was liaising with a Crisis Assessment Team over how to best handle a disturbed doctor.

As mentioned above, in requesting these changes in the new 1994 *Medical Practice Act*, the Board had anticipated additional benefits, especially hoping that ill and possibly impaired doctors would come forward earlier for help and treatment. We had underestimated the stigma associated with the Medical Practitioners Board, even a Board determined to be as helpful as possible to sick doctors. Within a couple of years, it was clear that we continued to have problems in regard to late presentation for help and in ensuring that sick doctors gained access to high quality care. The Board had no authority to play any role in rehabilitation and re-entry into practice. The Board began to discuss how we might be able to address these shortcomings.

A new way forward: the Doctors Health Program

The initiative of the New South Wales Medical Board to hold a joint conference of state and territory medical boards in 1991 indirectly led the Victorian Board to a way forward. The NSW joint conference opened up the Australian medical boards to regular contact with their North American counterparts. Through these contacts, especially through attendance at the annual conference of the Federation of American Medical Boards, Victorian Board members were able to learn at firsthand how impaired doctors were managed in other English-speaking jurisdictions. We noted especially the doctors' health services that had been gradually established in the USA and Canada that sought to promote early intervention and better care for such doctors. In 1994, many of these services had been established for 20–30 years. While there were some differences among them, they had in common the aim of encouraging doctors who were unwell and at risk of impairment to seek help, independently of the Medical Board, before their right to continue to practise was put in jeopardy.

The first formal discussion of a new way of doing things was in May 1995 when the Medical Practitioners Board of Victoria convened a one day meeting entitled the 'Impaired Practitioner Seminar'. Attendees included Board members, doctors who were involved in treating or assessing possibly impaired doctors, medical defence association lawyers and the two doctors who staffed the Victorian Doctors Health Advisory Service. Speakers included a representative of the NSW Medical Board who described their Board's approach and Dr Channa Wijesinghe, psychiatrist and then chair of the Health Committee of the Medical Practitioners Board. In Dr Wijesinghe's presentation, he described for the first time the broad outline of the Board's view as to what an independent 'impaired practitioners program' might look like. The seminar was successful in terms of bringing together stakeholders and people with expertise but did not lead to any decision as to what might be the next steps.

Following subsequent informal discussions among Board members, I prepared a discussion paper for the Board which canvassed the issues and made a recommendation for a new service to be established which would be independent of the Medical Practitioners Board and would provide expert help and support for ill doctors. The paper proposed that the service might be called the Victorian Doctors Health Institute and suggested that it might be useful if the service was in some way affiliated with a university faculty of medicine. Otherwise, the proposal was built around what were believed to be the best features of the North American programs. At a meeting of the Medical Practitioners Board, the broad thrust of what was proposed was endorsed by the Board, and I was authorised to undertake discussions with AMA Victoria.

The Chief Executive Officer of AMA Victoria, Dr Robyn Mason, was very supportive of the proposal but was aware that it may have been difficult to gain the full support of the Board of AMAV at that stage. The volunteer-based Victorian Doctors Health Advisory Service (DHAS), which was run under the auspices of AMAV, was a telephone service with advice provided by two experienced doctors, one of whom was a former President of AMAV. They shared all the on-call. As these doctors were nearing retirement from full-time clinical practice, AMAV was considering options as to how the DHAS would continue to provide services. A doctors' self-help group, Doctors in Recovery, was also at that stage discussing with AMAV options about service development and assistance. As a consequence, AMAV established a small working party to canvass future service models. It determined that the best long-term, sustainable and effective model was that offered by the Medical Practitioners Board proposal.

It was next decided by the Medical Practitioners Board, and with the strong support of the CEO of AMAV, that to move the concept ahead and hopefully gain the support of the Board of AMAV and others involved in matters concerning doctors health, another workshop of stakeholders should be held and that the Board should invite a medical director of a doctors' health program from one of the states of the USA to speak at the workshop. Funding such a visit would have been impossible without the financial independence afforded to the Medical Practitioners Board by the new 1994 *Medical Practice Act*. Equally importantly, finding a suitable person to invite from the USA would have been much more difficult without the personal contacts that had been established with our North American counterparts.

Through those contacts, an invitation was made to Dr Gerald Summer who was then the Medical Director of the Alabama Physician Health Program. We were well advised as Dr Summer was a very impressive speaker who had the additional credibility of coming to his job when a physical health issue led him to give up his private practice as a cardiologist. He was also deeply involved in the work of the US Federation of State Physician Health Programs so was able to describe the range of programs in place in the USA. He was the main speaker at our stakeholder workshop which was held at the premises of the Medical Practitioners Board in 1998. Our workshop was facilitated by Medical Board member, Dr Joanna Flynn. The stakeholders, numbering around 40 people, included members and senior staff of the Medical Practitioners Board, members of the Board of AMAV, the CEO of AMAV, and a number of Melbourne based doctors who were known to have a strong interest in doctors' health matters (these were mostly psychiatrists and many had acted as independent assessors for the Medical Practitioners Board).

It was an amazing meeting as from a position of some scepticism of many attendees at the outset, by the end of the evening there was unanimous support for a program akin to what was available in the USA and was being proposed by the Medical Practitioners Board. Armed with strong support of the medical profession via AMAV, the Board was then able to commence planning for the development of what was to be the Victorian Doctors Health Program. A planning committee was established with equal membership between the Medical Practitioners Board and AMAV. The members of the planning committee included Dr John Court and myself from the Medical Practitioners Board and Dr Robyn Mason and Dr Paul Woodhouse from AMA Victoria.

While the planning and the development of an agreed constitution and business plan was time-consuming, few obstacles were encountered during the 18–24 months of work. The then Minister for Health, Mr Rob Knowles, was supportive of the concept. This was vital as legal advice had indicated that, while the *Medical Practice Act* 1994 made the Board financially independent, the Act did not specifically authorise the Board to pay for such an arm's length independent service. Plans for the program were first announced to the medical profession and the public in January 2000. With the strong support of Minister Knowles and subsequently Minister John Thwaites, when the ALP came to power in late 1999, the Act was amended in May 2000 to enable the service to be established. The amendment meant that the Medical Practitioners Board could fully fund the new program from the fees collected each year for renewal of medical registration; thus, the program was to be funded by and hence effectively owned by all doctors in Victoria.

The next phase involved turning the concept into a reality. It was agreed that the new program would be set up as an incorporated company of which the MPBV and AMAV would be the joint owners and that the Program would be run by an independent Board of Directors. The crucial first step was to appoint the Board of Directors and a Chair of the Board. Under the constitution, the AMAV and the MPBV were each required to nominate two Board members (who could not be serving members of MPBV) and the two owners had to agree on an independent Chair of the Board. Dr Taffy Jones, an experienced, able and well-liked medical administrator was approached and he accepted the role of the inaugural Chair. The other inaugural Board members were Dr Sandra Hacker and Dr Paul Woodhouse (AMAV nominees) and Dr Channa Wijesinghe, who by now had retired from the Medical Practitioners Board, and Dr Doris Young (MPBV nominees).

There was much work to be done, especially by the Chairman. The constitution called for the establishment of a Consultative Council with nominees to come from the two (now three) medical schools, the medical colleges and several other organisations. All these organisations needed to be briefed on the establishment of VDHP, urged to support it, and asked to provide a nominee to the Consultative Council. To achieve this, Dr Jones visited all of them. The Consultative Council was to meet at least once a year; its purpose was to keep the Board of VDHP in close contact with the medical profession and to seek advice from the profession.

The new Board also needed to handle the transition from the long-established Doctors Health Advisory Service (DHAS) which had been run on an entirely voluntary basis and was available to help any doctor who had any sort of health problem. Some diplomacy was required to convince those who were running the DHAS that VDHP was aiming to provide a much more comprehensive and confidential service based on similar programs which had been running overseas for some time.

As one of the owners of the new service was the Medical Practitioners Board of Victoria, it was crucial to reassure all concerned that confidentiality for anyone attending VDHP would be absolutely guaranteed. To assist in providing this assurance, it was decided from the outset that the identity of individual clients of the service would not be known to members of the Board of Directors of VDHP.

The work of VDHP

VDHP aims included supporting the wellbeing of medical practitioners and medical students, through education and prevention, early intervention for those who are ill and/or at risk of becoming impaired, triage to best treatment (based on a detailed initial face to face assessment) and to high quality rehabilitation and, if needed, retraining to re-enter the workforce. VDHP provided support for participants and their families and sought to foster research into doctors' health. It provided training to support doctors to treat other doctors; and facilitation of a support group for some clients. The VDHP also offered to at-risk clients a voluntary case management program that could include random screening for drug use and identification of a workplace monitor. Case management has a long and mostly successful history in North America and has served the clients of VDHP well.

The VDHP Board appointed anaesthetist, Dr Jack Warhaft, as the inaugural medical director, commencing in February 2001. Dr Warhaft was a leading figure in the Doctors in Recovery organisation. The Board sent him on a short study tour of similar programs in Canada and the USA. An office manager and a clinical psychologist were also appointed and in May 2001 the program saw its first client.

In its fifteen years of existence, VDHP has become an essential support agency for medical students and medical practitioners. In 2015, there were 250 telephone enquiries and over 150 new face to face assessments (approximately 25% medical students, 50% doctors in training and 25% more senior doctors). Another 87 doctors and medical students were the recipients of ongoing support and/ or monitoring, which for some included workplace monitoring. In the difficult situation of doctors with substance use or drug dependence disorders, VDHP has published five-year outcomes of 80% return to work and freedom from drug use. In its first fifteen years, 1500 doctors and medical students were triaged by VDHP, representing approximately 7% of the Victorian medical workforce. Other core work has included extensive educational initiatives, preventive work with groups of medical students and doctors, 'doctors for doctors' workshops, and liaison with a wide range of agencies. Although there are other avenues of support for distressed medical students and doctors in training provided by medical schools and hospitals, the independence of VDHP is particularly attractive to these two groups. Until the advent of the national registration scheme in 2010, funding for VDHP was provided from the fees raised through annual renewal of medical registration; in current (2017) figures the service cost approximately 50 cents per week for every doctor in Victoria.

In late 2005, the inaugural Chairman of VDHP, Dr Taffy Jones, stepped down. I was invited by the owners of the VDHP, i.e. the Medical Practitioners Board and the Victorian AMA, to take over from him. A year later, the inaugural medical director who had done a good job in developing the service left VDHP. To keep the program running while we sought a new medical director, I was able to prevail on my longstanding friendship with Dr Greg Whelan, an addiction medicine expert and experienced clinician and administrator, who stepped into the breach as acting CEO, initially for 'a few months' that ran into well over a year.

The recruitment of a new medical director took some time as the position had to be advertised and interviews held, and then the successful applicant needed time to be free to take up the post. From a number of very good applicants, the selection committee chose Dr Kym Jenkins. Dr Jenkins had originally worked in general practice before training in psychiatry, and as a psychiatrist had worked as a liaison psychiatrist in a major general hospital where she had also established a support program for young trainees. This broad experience seemed to us to equip her perfectly for the task. She quickly settled into her role and did an outstanding job for the next ten years.

Dark clouds on the horizon

Unfortunately, during Dr Jenkins' time as medical director, dark clouds appeared on the horizon for VDHP, commencing in 2009 in the following way. The Council of Australian Governments (COAG) had set in train a process to replace state based registration and regulation of the health professions with a single national scheme. A task force was established to develop the national law for the system and to arrange the new regulatory framework. The task force gave several undertakings, many of which it failed to meet. One such undertaking was that the new system would incorporate the 'best' of what existed in the state-based systems. I naturally assumed that the new national law would provide a mechanism for continuing to fund VDHP.

I was dismayed when the first draft of the legislation was made available for public comment that funding for health programs had been omitted. As chair of the Board of VDHP, I arranged for the Medical Practitioners Board, AMA Victoria and VDHP to make a strongly worded joint submission urging that this oversight be corrected. The submission was copied to all state and territory health ministers. I also contacted counterpart organisations in South Australia and New South Wales, both of which received some funding from their respective state medical boards, urging them to make submissions. The next draft of the national law contained the desired wording, although expressed as an option and not an obligation.

Given the apparent reluctance at first to allow funding for programs like VDHP, I sensed that at the changeover to the national scheme, scheduled for July 2010, it was very unlikely that the new structure (i.e. the Medical Board of Australia) would be able to release funds immediately to keep VDHP afloat. On behalf of VDHP, I wrote to the Victorian Minister of Health, Mr Daniel Andrews, about the risk to the program and sought a meeting with him. It proved to be one of the best and shortest meetings I have ever had with a politician. He was clearly well-briefed and quickly informed me that he deemed VDHP (and the Victorian Nurses Health Program which had been established a little later) were vital organisations. The Minister assured me that full funding for VDHP was assured for three years from July 2010 and that this should give ample time for national funding to become available. I did not ask where the money was coming from. Later I was informed that the Minister had simply held back the necessary funds from the reserves of the Medical Practitioners Board that were due to be handed over to the Medical Board of Australia. So, a second threat to VDHP had been averted. Feeling happy about the future and having chaired the VDHP Board for five years, I decided to step down. The owners accepted my suggestion that Dr Robyn Mason take over as the new chair.

My confidence in the future for VDHP under the new national scheme proved to be short-lived. I watched and waited for the Medical Board of Australia to act on funding doctors' health services but nearly three years had elapsed without any action. I had kept in close contact with Robyn Mason and Kym Jenkins and I urged them to lobby the Victorian Health Minister, now Dr David Davies, a chiropractor. I was informed that, like his predecessor, Davies was a strong believer in the doctors and nurses health programs. He was able to raise this inertia at a meeting of state and territory health ministers and as a result, the health ministers directed the Medical Board of Australia to get on with it. The Medical Board now agreed as an interim measure to fund VDHP from the end of July 2013 when the Victorian funding agreement ended. Again, I felt that all would be well, only again to have my hopes dashed.

The Medical Board of Australia, for reasons never openly expressed, chose to provide funding that covered only approximately 65% of the annual budget of VDHP. As far as I can determine, the Medical Board of Australia's discomfort with full-funding of VDHP apparently arises from its belief that 'case management' should be restricted to the health committees of the state boards of the MBA. 'Case management' as used by VDHP refers to voluntary agreements with doctor clients that certain supportive elements will be put in place to assist their recovery and rehabilitation and includes such things as random testing for drugs, having a confidential monitor in the workplace, and regular attendance at a support group. The MBA seems to wish to equate case management with conditions placed on a doctor's registration, which of course can only be done by the MBA. In my view the MBA is confusing illness with impairment. Conditions on registration are only required where it is deemed that, without them, the doctor would pose a risk to the community. The MBA seems also to ignore the fact that a form of case management is already used in some areas of clinical practice: e.g. addiction medicine specialists may conduct breath tests for alcohol in their patients and some psychiatrists seek compliance with counselling through agreements that patients may be billed for failing to keep appointments without valid reason. There clearly is a grey zone wherein it can be difficult to decide whether a doctor should be managed and supported by either the Medical Board or by a health program. This grey zone is well-recognised and has been addressed by clear guidelines in Canadian and US jurisdictions and was the subject of an MOU between the MPBV and the VDHP.*

The VDHP could not survive at that level of funding without dismissing key staff and closing its ongoing support services for doctors in the program. It also became clear to me that the VDHP Board had no answers to this crisis. The Board's task was made more difficult through two factors. Dr Robyn Mason had resigned as Chair and a new chair was appointed. In law, the half ownership of VDHP had fallen to the Medical Board of Australia when it replaced the Medical Practitioners Board of Victoria in 2010. However, from where I sat, it seemed to me that the Medical Board of Australia was simply not interested in taking on any of the responsibilities that an owner was obliged to meet.

Finding additional sources of funding

Having a very strong personal interest in the future of VDHP, I decided to explore additional sources of funding. I knew the deans of two of the three medical schools in Victoria quite well and I was aware that increasingly the medical schools were referring medical students to VDHP

---

* For a more detailed discussion of this issue see: Breen, K J., 'Physician health and impairment in Australia: unsettled times', *Health Law Review* (Alberta), vol. 21, 2013: 23–8 and 'Disclosure of Physician Health Information: Seeking the right balance between confidentiality and public safety. Anonymous', *Health Law Review* (Alberta), vol. 21, 2013: 17–19.

and were very satisfied with the help provided. I soon ascertained that all three deans were happy to assist by providing funds to help bridge gaps over the next couple of years. Armed with this informal undertaking, I then was in a better position to approach two other organisations, the Victorian Medical Benevolent Fund and the Victorian Medical Insurance Agency, that were likely to be able to provide similar assistance and this proved to be the case. All of my negotiating had been done on an informal and personal basis without any authorisation of the VDHP Board. Now I needed to get that authorisation.

I requested that I attend a meeting of the Board of Directors and that request was granted. At the meeting, I outlined the informal discussions that I had held and recommended that the VDHP Board either grant me authority to formalise these discussions on the behalf of the Board or undertake the work itself. Although the Chair was clearly discomforted by my activities, his Board members strongly supported the granting of authority to me to negotiate on behalf of the Board. The negotiations were successfully completed and VDHP once again had a couple of years of breathing space. This was essential as the Medical Board of Australia was taking its time to decide what services were to be funded nationally.

In April 2014, the Medical Board announced that it would 'fund health programs to deliver a nationally consistent set of services to medical practitioners and students in all states and territories, to be run at arm's length from the Board'. However, in the meanwhile, it continued its deliberate underfunding of VDHP. I was concerned that the additional funds made available by the medical schools and the other two agencies were never seen as long-term propositions and wondered where other funds might come from. Given the increasing numbers of highly stressed junior doctors presenting to VDHP, it seemed to me that the Victorian Health Department might wish to help. But how could the Department be convinced?

Yet again, serendipity provided an opening. I play golf and, one Sunday morning early in 2015, I held a door open at my golf club for another golfer. It was Daniel Andrews, now the Premier of Victoria, also a keen golfer, who was visiting our club. He recognised me (from our one meeting in 2009!) and asked how VDHP was getting on. I chose not to speak in any detail but flagged my concerns in one sentence and offered to write to him. He indicated a willingness to receive a letter from me. That letter led to my meeting with a senior official in the Victorian Health Department. I was not involved in subsequent negotiations but the end result two years later was that the Health Department agreed on a long-term basis to make up the shortfall caused by underfunding from the Medical Board of Australia.

While negotiations with the Victorian Health Department were proceeding, the Medical Board of Australia finally put in place its chosen funding model in mid-2016. This had two serious flaws: the funding would come indirectly via a new company set up for this purpose by the federal Australian Medical Association, thereby diverting 10% of the funding away from clinical services; and the funding released still only met 65% of the budget of the tightly run Victorian program. As the Victorian Health Department had agreed to meet the shortfall, theoretically all should have been well. Sadly, yet another threat to the integrity of the program arose.

Another threat to the program

The original program when established in 2001 was jointly owned by the then Medical Practitioners Board of Victoria and the Victorian Branch of the Australian Medical Association and was run by an independent Board of Directors. The Medical Board of Australia, the successor in law to the Medical Practitioners Board of Victoria, declined a role as an owner. In late 2016, sole ownership was ceded to AMA Victoria, notionally to be held in trust for all doctors (only 30% of whom are thought to be AMA Victoria members). In mid-2017, that trust was severely threatened as the Board of Directors of the Health Program, now made up predominantly of persons nominated by AMA Victoria, decided to relocate the Program's office to AMA Victoria's headquarters in Parkville, against the advice of the staff of the Program. In becoming the sole owner of VDHP, the elected President of AMAV assumed chairmanship of the Board of VDHP. At the same time, the CEO of AMAV was appointed as CEO of VDHP, replacing the long-serving medical director who had served in this role. The relocation threatened a key element of the Program, namely assurance that attending the office of the Program offers maximum protection of confidentiality and privacy. The relocation raised possible issues of conflicts of interest around how the Program's funds, sourced from the medical profession and from the Victorian Government, were to be used. In protest at this relocation decision, three key staff members, including the experienced Medical Director, resigned. These resignations represented sixty percent of the Program's staff.

At the time of writing, calls had been made for AMA Victoria to reverse its decision on relocation, add truly independent directors to the Board of the Program and ensure that the Program is run for all Victorian doctors who are indeed the real owners of the Program. Calls were also made to the Victorian Health Department which now funds 35% of the Program to put pressure on AMA Victoria so these things happen. Unfortunately, this latest crisis took place at a time of increasing awareness of doctors' mental well-being, doctor suicides and concerns re mandatory reporting when the need for a truly independent and confidential doctors' health service such as VDHP had never been more crucial.

It remains deeply disappointing to me that the Medical Board of Australia appears to have taken a stance against VDHP and its comprehensive service. My disappointment is compounded by the fact that Dr Joanna Flynn, President of the Medical Board of Australia since it began in 2010, was the President of the Medical Practitioners Board of Victoria for several years and in that role presided over the launch of VDHP in 2001, soon after I had stepped down. As a member of the Medical Practitioners Board of Victoria she was, at my invitation, the facilitator of the workshop held in 1998 at which Dr Summer from the USA spoke and which workshop was the catalyst for the formation of VDHP.

Smouldering in the background and possibly still biasing the views of otherwise intelligent people are two past instances where case management was held to be a problem. The first instance was some unfortunate wording used in a sample case of a drug misusing doctor summarised on the VDHP website by the inaugural medical director many years ago which raised in the minds of some interstate readers that VDHP was 'hiding' troublesome doctors from the Medical Board. This of course was untrue as there was a memorandum of understanding in place between VDHP and the Medical Practitioners Board which was faithfully adhered to, there was regular contact between staff of VDHP and the health committee of the Board to discuss such problematic cases, and indeed, the Medical Practitioners Board was referring doctors to VDHP.

The second case which was of greater concern was the case of Dr James Latham Peters who eventually went to jail for infecting a large number of women with hepatitis C. From words spoken to me by a senior official in the Victorian Health Department in 2016, it was clear that VDHP had been apportioned some blame for the fact that Dr Peters, a known drug abusing doctor, was allowed to still be practising. This is incorrect. It is true that some years earlier Dr Peters had been a client of VDHP but at the time of his criminal conduct, he was under the supervision of the health committee of the Medical Practitioners Board of Victoria. In my view, it was unfortunate that the evidence in this regard was never made public in a court. Dr Peters pleaded guilty to the criminal charges so no evidence was called and the civil cases against him were settled out of court. My guess is that some of the negative attitudes to VDHP's use of case management can be explained by dissemination of this type of misinformation.

With the release of Medical Board funds to doctors health services in other states, hopefully these expanded services will be able in the future to achieve as much as has VDHP. In my experience sadly there exists a strange element in Australia of not wanting to learn from neighbouring states. Whether this reflects jealousy or insularity or some other influence I don't know. However, if the other states are reluctant to copy Victoria's lead in doctors' health matters, I sincerely hope that their leaders will visit North America to examine at first hand similar successful programs that have now been in place for forty years.

Chapter 7

SEXUAL MISCONDUCT BY DOCTORS

Under-reported and always harmful

During my time on the Medical Board, we dealt with a number of disturbing cases of sexual misconduct by doctors. I have already mentioned the case of the orthopaedic surgeon. The most grievous case was that of a Melbourne psychiatrist in his mid-forties who specialised in treating people with eating disorders. It was alleged that he had entered into sexual relationships with several young women he was supposedly helping. The psychiatrist presumably concluded that the evidence against him was overwhelming and damning. He chose not to attend the formal hearing that I chaired in 1996 and he was not legally represented. However, for the matter to proceed to a conclusion, the young women were required to give evidence on oath at an open hearing.

The women did not know each other. Their harrowing stories that they told under oath at the hearing were remarkably similar. Each had initially felt that the psychiatrist was a very good and caring doctor but gradually the nature of the relationship was changed to a personal one and then a sexual one. This seemed to be achieved through the doctor assuring the young patient that the social and sexual relationship was a vital part of therapy. The behaviour was eventually the subject of complaint as each patient realised how badly she had been mistreated, often in the setting where the psychiatrist wanted to end the sexual relationship. The emotional state of these unfortunate victims was very much what has been described by researchers around the world – their mental well-being had been made worse by the experience, they were clearly deeply traumatised, and they were likely to have great difficulty with the notion of ever trusting a doctor again.

Their evidence was overwhelming, the charges were found proven and the doctor was deregistered. I was very pleased with our 'reasons for decision' as it was intended to praise the enormous courage of the young women who came forward to give evidence in person to this public hearing. The content of our document was picked up by at least one reporter who wrote a very good summary of the case for the Melbourne *Age*.

There was a troubling antecedent to this case. Some four or five years earlier, the Board had received a complaint from the parents of their eighteen-year-old daughter who was attending the same psychiatrist for her eating disorder. The parents alleged that the doctor had taken their daughter on a weekend trip to southern New South Wales and they accused him of having an affair with their daughter. The Board regarded the allegations as very serious and set in train a formal disciplinary inquiry. However, as the date of the hearing drew closer, we were informed by the Board's solicitor that the eighteen-year-old patient of was not prepared to give evidence against the psychiatrist. The Board sought legal advice as to whether the Board had the power to subpoena the young woman and bring her to the planned hearing against her wishes. The legal advice was that this was not possible. The hearing lapsed and the psychiatrist went on with his appalling conduct unchecked. On reading a detailed report of the Board hearing in a Melbourne newspaper in 1996, the young woman concerned in the earlier aborted hearing telephoned the office of the Medical Practitioners Board to apologise for her refusal to give evidence. If she had given evidence then, several young women might have been saved from this predatory behaviour.

There are three common types of allegations of sexual misconduct received by medical boards. They are all distressing experiences for the victims but the most distressing is the conduct of the serial predator, usually a male psychiatrist, who uses the therapeutic relationship to seduce his patients. The second form is of a sole event of a sexual relationship that develops between a patient and a doctor. Again, usually the doctor is a male and the patient is female but the relationship may be homosexual and occasionally the doctor is female. There is often a scenario of a lonely middle-aged doctor entering a relationship with a willing current patient. Many such relationships may go unremarked as a complaint to the medical board is only likely if the doctor breaks off the relationship. The third common form of complaint and allegation is in the field of what are called 'sexually intrusive examinations' i.e. breast and or genital examinations. In these instances, the patient alleges that the examination was conducted for improper purposes, i.e. for the sexual pleasure of the doctor. All these forms of professional conduct are unethical, wrong and harmful.

Sexual misconduct is worryingly common. One US report gives a figure of thirteen percent of doctors admitting to sexual contact with patients, most describing involvement with several patients. In a questionnaire study that over three hundred Australian psychiatrists responded to, the figure was 7.6%. More recently another Australian study reported that sexual misconduct was the most frequent cause of deregistration of doctors in Australia. I am sure that the problem remains under reported in Australia despite the introduction of mandatory reporting in 2010.

The barriers to reporting are powerful. Victims are reluctant to come forward to complain, knowing that if they go through with their complaint their evidence will be strenuously tested in a public hearing. The commonest scenario is a female patient of a male psychiatrist who has been misled into a sexual relationship in part because of vulnerability (many are vulnerable because of a past history of childhood sexual abuse and subsequent uncertainty about sexual boundaries) and in part because the all-powerful doctor has misused what should be a strong therapeutic relationship. When the patient finally realises the abuse, most often after being rejected, there are often confused feelings of guilt and self-blame as well as feelings of powerlessness to take action. There is an extensive literature on this subject for any reader who is seeking more information.*

* An excellent starting point is the book by Dr Peter Rutter entitled *Sex in the Forbidden Zone. When Men in Power Abuse Women's Trust*, Harper Collins, London, 1995. Another source of a summary of the international literature can be found in Ch. 12 entitled *Sexual and*

Seeking to do better in Victoria

Through reports of the Board's investigating officers and via sitting on and chairing panels which conducted hearings into sexual misconduct allegations, I became very aware of the enormous emotional strain placed on those who might wish to make allegations. I felt that the Medical Board needed to do more to reduce this and other barriers and to explore whether there were ways to reduce the occurrence of such offences. The Medical Board agreed to set up working party to look at these matters. Board member, Dr Kay Leeton, an obstetrician and gynaecologist, agreed to chair the working party. In the first year of the life of the working party, Dr Leeton had some difficulties in that two male board members seemed to want to minimise the problems of sexual misconduct. In addition, both behaved in a manner which suggested they were chauvinists. She bravely stared them down, and her committee made some major progress, researching the topic, producing new guidelines and seeking to stimulate more open reporting by other doctors who learn of such allegations. Her group also tried to raise interest in the topic with other professions including psychology and religion.

To try to move the sexual misconduct debate along in Victoria, we invited Dr Gary Johnson, who had played a central role in changes in Ontario in Canada, which had included the requirement of mandatory reporting of allegations, to visit Melbourne. By this time, I had got to

---

other boundaries in our textbook *Good Medical Practice: Professionalism, Ethics and Law* published by the Australian Medical Council in 2016.

know Gary quite well through attending Canadian and international meetings and he came willingly. He spoke very well to a couple of different audiences. His visit led to a brief flurry of activities which have since died down. In the late 1990s, the Medical Practitioners Board did raise with government the need for a change to the Medical Act to bring in mandatory reporting and also raised the concept that doctors who wished to notify the Board of sexual misconduct allegations be given some legal protection. These changes finally arrived nationally in 2010.

One initiative that arose from Dr Leeton's working party was the recruitment of a female legally qualified investigating officer to handle these cases and we were fortunate to find Ms Lisa Walker who not only was a lawyer but also had a degree in psychology. There is no data to support my contention but I am sure that her work made the stress experienced by complainants considerably easier for them to cope with.

The Board still had the issue of seeking to minimise the stress involved for complainants giving their evidence at public hearings. Via a serendipitous meeting, I came up with the idea of establishing a Board 'Support Service'. By this time, I had become quite close to Professor Vernon Plueckhahn because of our work on the Professional Practice Program. At one of our meetings at the Victorian Institute for Forensic Medicine, possibly over our textbook, he introduced me to Ms Carmel Benjamin and explained to me that Ms Benjamin had very recently stepped down as the head, and founder, of a volunteer support service for distressed people who needed to appear before the Victorian law courts. She had been awarded an AM for this highly original initiative.

Luckily, I was able to convince Ms Benjamin that she might like to help the Medical Board establish a similar service. This soon came into being, conducted by her and an experienced colleague. It was made available both to those making complaints or allegations of misconduct and to doctors facing disciplinary actions and was fully funded by the Medical Board. In negotiating the setting up of this initiative, the Board needed and obtained the understanding of the medical indemnity organisations, as it could readily have been misconstrued as a service designed just to support complainants. I believe it served a very valuable purpose. It was not restricted to sexual misconduct cases. The service was used more by complainants than by doctors, as most doctors attending hearings to answer allegations of serious misconduct already felt well-supported by their medical indemnity organisation.

As far as I know the service was later abandoned, possibly because hearings of serious misconduct allegations were taken out of the hands of the Medical Practitioners Board and passed to the Victorian Civil and Administrative Tribunal in around 2007. Perhaps that tribunal might consider re-establishing a similar service.

Even today, I doubt that most members of the medical profession and the legal profession really understand the harm that results from sexual misconduct. That harm not only involves individual patients but also harm to the confidence that the community needs to have in its doctors. I also believe that the medical profession, and most notably one subsection, psychiatry, has not done enough to try to minimise the problem or deter potential offenders. I recall with dismay a hearing that I was involved in. A middle-aged recently divorced male general practitioner was alleged to have had an affair with a female patient he was treating for depression. He was found guilty and as both a penalty and for general deterrence, his registration was suspended for six months. He appealed the decision to the Victorian Supreme Court. The single judge hearing the case (who we were told was about to retire) did not overrule the guilty finding but reduced the penalty to a reprimand. In my view, the judge was telling our community that it was not a serious issue for a doctor to use his practice to establish a sexual relationship with a patient, one who through her illness was vulnerable.

Chapter 8

THE AUSTRALIAN MEDICAL COUNCIL

Its role in examining and accrediting

The history of the first twenty-five years of the Australian Medical Council (AMC) was published in 2010.* I had the good fortune to be a very small part of that history. The AMC arose from the need to 'repatriate' the role of the UK General Medical Council which had up until the late 1980's accredited Australia's medical schools for the purposes of registration by Australia's medical boards. While accreditation of Australian medical schools by UK General Medical Council might seem like a colonial remnant, it lasted a long time because it served a useful secondary purpose for many Australian doctors as it meant that registration to practise in the UK was automatically assured.

The AMC was established as an incorporated body based in Canberra in 1985, with a majority of the Council membership being the eight presidents of the State and Territory Medical Boards. Thus, when I was appointed as President of the Medical Practitioners Board of Victoria in 1994, I automatically became a member of the AMC.

* *Assuring Medical Standards; The Australian Medical Council 1985–2010,* (ed.) Geffen L. ISBN 978-1-875440-72-6.

I served on the AMC initially under the presidency of Dr John Horvath, whom I knew from my time spent as a trainee physician at the Royal Prince Alfred Hospital in Sydney in 1969 and 1970. When Dr Horvath stepped down in 1997, it was assumed that the then deputy AMC president, Dr Ross Kalucy, President of the South Australian Medical Board, would be elected President. However, Dr Kalucy declined the nomination and at the last minute I was asked to nominate and was elected unopposed. By then, the AMC processes for accrediting our medical schools and for examining overseas trained doctors were well established, so the expected role of the incoming President was pretty much to assist in keeping these well-oiled processes running. The chances of being a reformist in such a national body are very slim.

Hunger-striking doctors

One burning issue at the time was political agitation by some overseas trained doctors (OTDs) protesting that the AMC examination standard was too high and that this had been artificially set to exclude overseas graduates. Some OTDs had been on a hunger strike in Sydney during 1997. They had earlier gained some sympathy from the Human Equal Rights and Opportunity Commission (HREOC, but now known as the Australian Human Rights Commission) and had initially won a case alleging discrimination against an OTD. This was not a case we could win in the court of public opinion, even though we were confident that the educational standards set were quite fair, that most OTDs were passing the examination and that the agitators had appalling knowledge of medicine. We simply had to let the case run its course, which included the AMC successfully appealing the HREOC decision to the High Court. It was not long after this that the Federal Government changed the legislation such that HREOC could no longer hold its own inquiries and instead had to take cases to the Federal Court. I wondered how much the overstepping of the mark and taking sides with a small group of vocal OTDs, had contributed to the 'clipping of the wings' of HREOC.

At that time, politicians of all persuasions saw an opportunity to criticise medical boards and the AMC under the guise of attacking doctors protecting their own positions. It is amusing to see how quickly the political wheel has turned especially following the saga of Dr Jayant Patel ('doctor death') in Bundaberg in Queensland.* Now the medical board and the AMC are criticised for not being strict enough in assessing OTDs! Dr Patel was eventually exonerated of manslaughter charges but was deregistered for other reasons including his many clinical failings. While he probably should never have been registered to practise medicine in Australia and should not have been undertaking major surgery at Bundaberg, in my view he also became a scapegoat for the failings of the health system in Queensland.

The HREOC case had one accidental positive outcome for the AMC. As part of the court case, the AMC was obliged to release its large bank of multiple choice examination questions. This of course undermined the security of the examination process and the questions could not be used again. It caused a lot of additional work creating a new bank of questions. Following a suggestion by Professor Vernon

---

* https://en.wikipedia.org/wiki/Jayant_Patel.

Marshall, chair of the AMC examinations committee, this negative was turned into a positive. The AMC assembled an editorial group led by Professor Marshall and created an excellent educational book for examination candidates based around the released questions. *Annotated Multiple Choice Questions*, by Marshall VC, Clark AL, Buzzard AJ et al and published by Blackwell Publishing Melbourne in 1997 was very well received by candidates. This was the start of a concerted effort by the AMC to publish other educational material which has included an *Anthology of Medical Conditions* and a *Handbook of Clinical Assessment*.

Opportunity for reforms

To my surprise, in my role as President, it was not long before an opportunity for positive reforms arrived in the AMC mail in the form of a letter from then Federal Health Minister, Dr Michael Woolridge, inviting the AMC to consider taking on a new role. For many years Australia had a national committee for the recognition of medical specialities. It was dominated by the existing medical specialist colleges and had obtained a reputation for blocking newly emerging medical specialties. The anger created by such actions had a lot more to do with money than with status, since recognised specialists were rewarded with larger rebates for their fees from Medicare. Michael Woolridge's letter invited the AMC to take over this role and also invited the AMC to suggest ways of improving the system.

The letter was enthusiastically received, especially by me. I had shared the experience of the Victorian Medical Board in the mid-1980s of dealing with a doctor who had established a new specialist medical college and who was accused of breaching advertising regulations. It had occurred to me then that, just as medical schools needed to be externally accredited so that the community could have faith in their graduates, so too should all medical colleges, old or new, be externally accredited. I mentioned this notion at a Medical Board meeting at that time and I was quite surprised at how negatively it was received by my colleagues. I think some members even laughed. Now some ten or more years later, the letter from the Minister opened the door widely to such a concept. The story is told in the history of the first 25 years of the AMC,* so I will omit the full details.

I chaired a working party which had the task of developing a response to the request of Dr Woolridge. The working party brought together the existing medical colleges and the medical boards and this group's work resulted in the setting up of two new AMC processes. We were enormously helped by two community/consumer members added to the working party, on John Horvath's recommendation. They were Ms Kate Moore and Ms Annabel Bennett. Ms Moore had recently stepped down from her position as CEO of the Consumers Health Forum while Ms Bennett was a lawyer who held a PhD in biochemistry and had served on health registration boards (and later became a judge of the Federal Court and served as Chair of the NHMRC and Chancellor of Bond University). Their contributions through bringing a consumer and community perspective to our deliberations proved critical in what was achieved, especially in convincing

---

* See ch. 5 in *Assuring Medical Standards; The Australian Medical Council 1985–2010*, (ed.) Geffen L. ISBN 978-1-875440-72-6.

the more conservative leaders of the medical colleges of the potential benefits of external accreditation.

One of those processes was the establishment of a new AMC committee to assess applications for the recognition of new medical specialties and to advise the Federal Health Minister regarding access to Medicare benefits. The second was the establishment of a committee for the external accreditation of the training programs offered by new and existing medical colleges on a five to ten year accreditation cycle. The latter process has led to significant improvements in the training and examination processes of the medical colleges.

One internal reform that I played a part in was to restructure and rename the AMC Uniformity Committee. The committee had existed since the Council was formed. Its purpose was to promote uniformity of medical registration and other board processes between the eight state and territory medical boards. This was probably an impossible aim as the committee had no effective means of influencing the state-based legislation that guided medical registration. The membership of the Uniformity Committee included the eight medical board presidents together with two or three other members of the Council. It met at least once a year. In my time as a member, it seemed to have no focus and little work to do. It did allow some board presidents to complain bitterly about 'Canberra'. The members who were not board presidents found that any attempt to raise differences between jurisdictions that might benefit from attention fell on deaf ears. Some board presidents resented the presence of these committee members and felt that they did not understand the work of medical boards. Those board presidents began to argue that what was needed was a committee of medical board presidents that was separate from the AMC. I felt that splitting away from the AMC in such a way would serve little purpose and instead suggested that the AMC constitution be amended to limit membership of the committee to the board presidents and to drop the name 'Uniformity'. This change was accepted by Council and the committee was renamed the Joint Medical Boards Advisory Committee.

Peace reigned but little changed in my time. Later the Committee embraced the concept that the AMC, together with the medical boards, would develop a national code of conduct for all doctors in Australia. By that time several Australian medical boards had issued codes of conduct of varying quality and usefulness. The process was supported by a grant from the Federal Department of Health and the end result was the document known as 'Good Medical Practice: a code of conduct for doctors in Australia'. In 2010, this code was adopted by the new Medical Board of Australia.

Proposing a single national registration body

I was far less successful with another notion that I raised with the AMC and the medical board presidents. In 1995 or thereabouts, the AMC held a two-day retreat for the purpose of reviewing its work and to plan for the future. Various AMC members were asked to speak to selected topics. My topic was the relationship between the AMC and the state and territory medical boards. As this was a retreat, no idea was banned from being raised. At this time, the AMC, with the medical boards, had negotiated a process of mutual recognition of medical registration between jurisdictions as a means of making interstate movement of doctors simpler. The medical boards had cooperated with the AMC to allow the AMC to house a 'national compendium of medical registers'.

I felt that these developments could well lead eventually to a single national registration body, i.e. a national medical board, and if this was so, then the existing boards would be wise to embrace the idea in order to achieve a workable outcome. I did not put a lot of work into my talk but I did take the trouble to arrange a meeting with the chairman of the Australian Stock Exchange. I was aware that the national stock exchange had arisen from existing state-based stock exchanges and I wondered if I could learn from the leadership of the Australian Exchange how this all came about. The chairman and one of his senior people generously gave me an hour of their time but we seemed to come from different worlds and I gained very little. In my talk at the retreat, I proposed that the state and territory medical boards should proactively seek to merge as one national board with eight branches, under the umbrella of the AMC. My idea had not been thought through and not surprisingly, it gained no interest or support from the other seven board presidents. Looking back, I now think that, if any of them had imagined that within fifteen years we would be saddled with a national medical board and a separate national regulator under a flawed system, we might have had a valuable discussion.

I enjoyed my time with the AMC although I found chairing Council meetings quite stressful. Council then was made up of the eight state and territory medical board presidents and senior people representing the medical colleges, the medical schools, the Australian Medical Association and the Federal Department of Health. There were some very powerful egos around the table and some deeply vested interests. The attitudes of the presidents of the medical boards of the smaller states tended to be conservative. Linked to a sense of paranoia about 'Canberra', this made for a recipe for obstruction to most change. However, in my early time on Council, I had stood up for 'states' rights sufficiently loudly that even the most conservative of the other medical board presidents seemed to trust me. I was impressed by the professionalism of the AMC staff and became, and have remained, very friendly with the CEO, Mr Ian Frank, his deputy, Ms Theanne Walters, and senior staff member, Ms Susan Buick.

Learning from other countries: the international association

I was always interested in learning from other countries in every field in which I worked. The tendency of Australia, and indeed most English-speaking nations, to turn only to other English-speaking countries for example or inspiration is something I find depressing. I encountered a typical example of this blinkered view in one group of doctors which particularly astounded me when I was on sabbatical leave in France in 1980. I had travelled to the UK to attend a meeting of the British Society of Gastroenterology. At the conference dinner, I sat with about ten or so British gastroenterologists who asked me what I was doing there. Collectively they seemed disbelieving that I could actually be learning something new from the French and were oblivious to the outstanding work of the liver specialists at Beaujön Hospital in Paris.

In 1994, soon after I had taken over as Medical Board President, I attended an AMC meeting where I learned that the American medical regulators had convened a meeting in Washington on international approaches to the regulation of the medical profession. In typical American tendency to hyperbole, this small conference, attendance at which was by invitation only and to which only seven nations had been invited, was called the 'First International Conference on Medical Regulation'. It may have been the first but it was barely international as the only nations invited were English-speaking. The conference was to be 'back-to-back' with the annual meeting of the US Federation of State Medical Boards.

By the time I went to that AMC meeting, the Australian delegation had been chosen. I had already made plans to visit the US at around that time to examine some hospitals in another role that I had at St Vincent's Hospital, Melbourne, so I arranged to be in Washington and invited myself to the conference. With a few others, I sat in rows at the back as 'observers'. At the end of the meeting, Australia's offer to host the second such conference in two years' time was accepted. Back home, I felt that it was likely that John Horvath as AMC President would want the conference to be held in his home city of Sydney and I was very surprised when he suggested that it be held in Melbourne. I found myself as convenor of the organising committee for the 1996 'Second International Conference on Medical Regulation'.

It is a long story but suffice it to say that the organising committee was able to turn the second conference into a truly international conference open to any nation and that twenty nations sent delegates. One of the most illuminating invited speakers was a medical regulator from Sweden where their system is very different from the systems common to English speaking countries. The program committee made one planning decision that it came to regret. Keen not to lose money on the conference, it was decided to open the conference to any doctors interested in medical regulation. By doing this, the attendance was enhanced to around 200 registrants. Among them was a small group of disgruntled Australian-based overseas trained doctors (OTDs) who were highly critical of the examinations conducted by the Australian Medical Council. As mentioned above, some OTDs had taken the Council to the Human Rights and Equal Opportunity Commission (and later held hunger strikes in Sydney). We had not anticipated that some among them might use the Second International Conference to make further protests. They did this by seeking to harangue the Victorian Minister for Health at the welcome cocktail party, requiring prompt action on the part of the organising committee. Two of their number asked questions at one of the panel discussions during the conference but, as the questions were not relevant to the subject matter, all that was achieved was some puzzlement among the international attendees.

At the Washington conference in 1994, the UK General Medical Council sent representatives but seemed not to engage deeply in the event. I suspect this related to their sense that as the General Medical Council is over 150 years old, the UK could claim to have 'invented' medical regulation and were miffed that their American cousins had stolen a march on them. They later sent delegates to the Melbourne conference, including their new President, Sir Donald Irvine, and their new Registrar, Mr Finlay Scott. I did not warm to Sir Donald but I warmed to Finlay Scott immediately and we later worked together to good effect.

My personal antipathy to Irvine's style, which to me appeared patrician by Australian standards, may have clouded my assessment of his contributions and those of the UK GMC. He came to his position with the GMC at a time of a crisis of confidence in the UK medical profession and in self-regulation of the profession, emanating from events and people including the Bristol Hospital scandal and the conduct of murderous Dr Shipman. Undoubtedly change was needed and some of those changes required clearly articulated documents which the GMC had issued. However, Irvine seemed unaware that the problems faced by the UK medical profession were not universal beyond the UK. Indeed, I believe that those were problems stored up by the UK class system, a paternalistic attitude of many of its doctors, and the sense that the medical profession could never be wrong. The notion of patient autonomy came very late to the UK and perhaps has not completely arrived even now. As the UK health care system offers little by the way of choice, patients have few options but to accept the status quo.

Irvine seemed to feel that because his GMC had created useful guidelines for the dilemmas faced in Britain, other countries should be grateful and should adopt these as international guidelines. He later used his powerful position as president or immediate past president of the GMC to promote his ideas quite widely. Even the editor of the *Medical Journal of Australia* was taken in by his notions. Rather than seek ideas from within Australia, the *Medical Journal of Australia* reproduced Irvine's papers, assuming that they were directly relevant here. Within the UK, Irvine's successor as President of the GMC had to battle the public relations machine of a health care organisation in which Irvine based himself, named the 'Picker Institute Europe'.* This name suggested a pan-European base but the web site at that time showed a board of directors drawn mostly from the UK with one or two from the USA.

The British seem to have a very odd way of handing out titles. I came to realise that when the GMC is about to install a newly elected President, the government of the day arranges for him (I don't think that there has yet been a woman president) to be awarded a knighthood, before any service has been rendered to the community via the GMC. This occurred with Sir Donald Irvine and with his successor, Professor Sir Graeme Catto, but the practice seems to have lapsed more recently.

At our 1996 Melbourne conference, a group of representatives of the seven nations who had been at the first conference met to discuss the idea of forming an international association of medical regulatory agencies. I found it amusing and instructive to observe the obvious jockeying for status between the UK and the USA delegates. We agreed to form a steering committee and thus I found myself working with Finlay Scott and some other very fine people, particularly a couple of Canadians, especially Dr Dale Dauphinee, the CEO of the Medical Council of Canada, who in his earlier life had also been a gastroenterologist.

* http://www.picker.org/.

121

Representing smaller countries, the Australian and Canadian delegates over the next few years found ourselves as 'honest brokers' or peacemakers between these two larger countries, the USA and the UK. By working together we could quietly enlist the voting numbers from our Irish, New Zealand and South African colleagues (all ex-colonials like us!). Finlay Scott proved to be an adept and flexible negotiator. At a critical meeting of the steering group which was held in Victoria on Vancouver Island in British Columbia, Canada in 1999, the chair was scheduled to be the UK. Sir Donald Irvine could not attend so Finlay Scott chaired the meeting and chaired it brilliantly. He knew from discussions with the delegates of the smaller countries that if he needed to call for votes on such issues as the draft constitution or the name of the new association that he had the numbers.

The argument over the proposed name was a diversion but emphasised how the Americans think, in that they wanted a more grandiose title of something like the 'World Federation of Medical Boards'. It was not possible to politely point out that this was 'over the top' in that we had no authority to call ourselves a 'world' anything, so I argued instead that Australia could readily join an 'association' but if we went down the 'federation' path, we might have to seek government approval. This was an argument made up on the spur of the moment on my part. I had no idea if it was true. However, the point was accepted and the steering committee decided on the more low-key name of 'International Association of Medical Regulatory Agencies' (IAMRA). The committee also reached a compromise between the UK and the USA delegates in that neither nation took the inaugural chairmanship; instead it went to Canada.

I attended the third international conference in Cape Town in 1998 and the fourth in Oxford in 2000. After I left the AMC in 2000, I have since observed from a distance the continued growth of IAMRA. I did attend two more of their international conferences, on each occasion as an invited speaker. One was in Toronto, Canada in 2002 and the other in Wellington, New Zealand in 2006.

In both instances, the program committee wanted me to address topics which had strong ethical themes. In Toronto, I gave a paper on research misconduct. This was stimulated by my interest in the manner in which doctors who were alleged to have engaged in research misconduct seemed to be handled differently among the various jurisdictions. As mentioned, in the UK, the GMC was very active in 'prosecuting' such allegations. By contrast, in the USA, serious proven offences seemed to be ignored by the state medical boards. In Australia, we had a mixed record. The NSW Medical Board and the NSW Medical Tribunal had dealt with allegations of research misconduct against the discoverer of thalidomide toxicity, Dr William McBride, and in Victoria in the 1980s, we had dealt with the case of Dr Ashoka Prasad, an Indian doctor who was later demonstrated to be a serial fabricator. But in general, Australian medical boards seemed to not be involved in research misconduct matters.

In reviewing the international literature on research misconduct, the most amazing account that I came across was about an American surgeon working for the British Army during the First World War who claimed to have invented a new imaging device for assessing internal injuries, which he called a 'delineator'. The device was soon found to be a fake, he was subjected to a court martial and sentenced to death. The death penalty was later commuted and he died in prison. The talk I gave in Canada I later turned into a paper published locally in the *Internal Medicine Journal** and I have since used my knowledge of this area in some work for the National Health and Medical Research Council. At the Toronto meeting, I was deeply honoured when my Canadian colleagues made a presentation to me of a framed award acknowledging my work in helping establish IAMRA.

During the 1990s and early 2000s, I had the pleasure of visiting Canada on a number of occasions for meetings with medical regulators and later with people working in the area of the ethics of medical research. The Medical Practitioners Board of Victoria invited two very impressive Canadians to Australia to assist the Board in some of its work. In all of these dealings, I found that the people were a pleasure to work with and that Canadians and Australians have a great deal in common. I also found that those working in medical regulation in Canada were forward looking and innovative with much that Australia could learn from. Although I was never personally or directly involved, the examinations arm of Australian Medical Council developed a close collaboration with its Canadian counterpart to the mutual benefit of both countries.

In Wellington, I chose as my theme the topic of 'medical professionalism' and took aim at those who felt that the problems facing the medical profession in the USA, Canada and parts of Europe could be solved through a new approach to professionalism and a new 'social contract' with

---

* Breen, K J, 'Misconduct in medical research: whose responsibility?', *Internal Medicine Journal*, vol. 33, 2003: 186–91.

the community. I argued that the 'social contract' described was unusual in that there had been no consultation with the communities concerned. I also argued that the problems were not due to any lack of professionalism but could be traced to a failure of the medical profession in many countries to acknowledge and adjust to profound changes in health care, changes that had altered the balance of the application of ethical principles in daily medical practice.[†] I was very pleased with the positive response that my talk received. It was after this talk that some UK GMC delegates aired their concerns with me over the contrary 'universalist' stance taken by their immediate past president, Sir Donald Irvine.

IAMRA has continued to grow in terms of membership numbers, reaching 111 member organisations from 48 countries in 2017.[‡] I am not sure what it has achieved or might still achieve in the future. If one wished to be very negative, one might say that it has contributed to bringing the possibility of the UK revalidation process to Australia and in this and other ways, might be speeding the process of over-regulation of the medical profession. It has also provided a forum for the new national regulator, the Australian Health Practitioner Regulation Agency (see Chapter 14), to promote its credentials to delegates from unsuspecting nations.

---

† Breen, K J, 'Medical professionalism – is it really under threat?', *Medical Journal of Australia,* vol. 186, 2007: 596–8.
‡ http://www.iamra.com/.

Chapter 9

ANOTHER TURNING POINT

Appointment to the Australian Health Ethics Committee

My appointment as a member of the Australian Health Ethics Committee (AHEC) in 1997 was hardly serendipitous and was not a huge surprise, although it was not an appointment that I sought. Dr Bernard Neal, recently retired from presidency of the Medical Board of Victoria, was appointed a member of AHEC for the 1995–7 triennium under the category of a member 'with knowledge of the regulation of the medical profession'. I was thus aware of the committee but was not across its key functions. Membership is renewed every three years, as the entire NHMRC works on a triennial appointment system. I was not approached by anyone but apparently my name was put forward for the 1997–2000 triennium by one of the nominating bodies. At the time, our text book, *Ethics, Law and Medical Practice*, had just been published so this, together with my long experience as a member and now President of the Medical Practitioners Board of Victoria, may have made me a suitable candidate for the same category of membership as Dr Neal. I was offered appointment and I accepted it. By now, I had resigned from my full-time appointment at St Vincent's Hospital and was working there on a limited sessional basis as well as conducting a very small private medical practice. I felt that I should be able to fit in this work on AHEC with my continuing roles on the Medical Practitioners Board and the Australian Medical Council.

The Australian Health Ethics Committee is a committee of the National Health and Medical Research Council (NHMRC). Although the NHMRC dates back to 1937, AHEC was only established when the new *National Health and Medical Research Council Act* (*NHMRC* Act 1992) was passed by the Federal Parliament in 1992. In very informal terms AHEC can be described as Australia's national bioethics committee. It replaced the short-lived National Bioethics Consultative Committee, a brave committee which may have doomed itself by being more adventurous than our politicians wanted. AHEC, as its replacement, was given narrower terms of reference but it was also given a very effective means of assuring a membership with a broad base.

Those terms of reference were identified in the *NHMRC* Act 1992 as three functions: (a) to advise the NHMRC on ethical issues relating to health; (b) to develop and give the NHMRC guidelines for the (ethical) conduct of medical research involving humans; and (c) such other functions as the Minister from time to time determines. (The last term of reference was amended in 2006 to read 'any other functions conferred on the Committee in writing by the Minister after consulting the CEO'.)

Under the *NHMRC Act* 1992, the membership of AHEC totalled fifteen people, in categories that included persons with expertise in medical ethics, law, philosophy and religion, and others with experience in various subfields of health research, medical practice, nursing, health consumer issues, disability issues and a person with expertise in the regulation of the medical profession. The relevant Federal Minister (the Minister of Health) was obliged to seek nominees from a number of peak national bodies and those bodies were required to provide three names for consideration in the relevant category of membership. At that time, in appointing both the chair of AHEC and the member of AHEC with expertise in medical ethics, the Federal Health Minister was obliged to seek approval from the state and territory health ministers.

I attended my first meeting with some anxiety as I feared that I would be sitting alongside people with much more knowledge of medical ethics and the ethics of medical research than I had. That anxiety was well-based but because of the quality of the members, good chairmanship, and my eventual discovery that discussing ethical issues did not need a strong theoretical knowledge base, I soon felt comfortable and was enjoying the work. I did not play a very active role in the work of AHEC in those early years. I was not part of its executive committee that met by telephone between infrequent face to face meetings of the whole committee. I was not involved in a working party that was asked to produce an urgent report to the Federal Minister of Health on the ethics of human cloning, a request triggered by the dramatic announcement in 1996 of the cloning of 'Dolly' the sheep in Scotland. And I missed parts of a couple of meetings because of clashes with commitments as a member of the Australian Medical Council.

Building up future trouble

However, I participated fully in regularly reviewing the progress being made on a key national document and product of AHEC, the *National Statement on Ethical Conduct in Research Involving Humans* (the *National Statement*), which after approval by the NHMRC, was issued in 1999. There were tensions around the AHEC table as this document was being finalised. I sensed that we were building up future trouble for the committee but did not fret too much as I was not planning to seek re-appointment at the end of my three years.

The potential trouble unfolded thus. Under its legislation, AHEC was charged with developing the *National Statement*. The *NHMRC Act* made it clear that the Council had to accept the document or reject it; i.e. the Council could not amend it. Furthermore, as the remit of the NHMRC clearly is restricted to 'health and medical research', the *National Statement* was focussed on these areas of human research. The stakeholders consulted in two rounds of public consultation during its development were restricted to those involved in health and medical research. Very late in its development, the chair of AHEC, an academic lawyer, actively pursued a suggestion that it would be good if the *National Statement* were to apply more widely to all types of research involving humans and as a result several key agencies became official endorsers of the new document. The agencies included the Australian Vice-Chancellors Committee (now known as Universities Australia), the Australian Research Council, the Australian Academy of the Humanities, the Australian Academy of Science and the Academy of Social Sciences in Australia.

Not unexpectedly, several of these agencies, having read the document that they were being asked to endorse, requested last minute alterations to some of the text. The chair found himself with an AHEC whose members refused to accept most of these changes. This refusal was not petty but was based on a desire that the protection of human subjects involved in medical research not be diminished. It was also based on the need for the final document to accurately reflect the extensive public consultation that had been undertaken.

When the *National Statement* was released in 1999, many rank and file researchers in fields outside health and medical research were quick to complain that they had never been consulted over the content of the document and to point out (correctly in my view) that there are sections of the document that could not be readily applied to their fields of research. Apart from this unhappiness, the document was very well received by the over 200 Human Research Ethics Committees across the nation and by health and medical researchers generally. The unhappiness of the non-health researchers was left to simmer until the next revision of the *National Statement*, required in five years' time.

Human Research Ethics Committees, originally called Institutional Ethics Committees, became a requirement for research funding by the NHMRC in 1973. Their role is to prospectively assess and where appropriate approve research proposals according to the *National Statement*. Their membership as provided for in the *National Statement* includes an independent chairperson; at least two lay people, one man and one woman, who have no affiliation with the institution and do not currently engage in medical, scientific, legal or academic work; at least one person with knowledge of, and current experience in, the professional care, counselling or treatment of people; at least one person who performs a pastoral care role in a community; at least one lawyer; and at least two people with current research experience that is relevant to research proposals being considered. In large institutions, the committees carry a big workload and all committees take on a very responsible task. This work is usually performed on an honorary basis although commercially based fee for service HRECs have also been established in recent years.

Two other initiatives were begun towards the end of my first three years as a member of AHEC. They were both to cause problems for the next AHEC and its chair. Both were handled by the AHEC executive committee and I had no role in either matter. The first was a decision taken by AHEC and agreed to by the NHMRC that a handbook for human research ethics committees was to be commissioned. The handbook was intended to assist human research ethics committee members in interpreting and applying the new *National Statement*. Expressions of interest were called for and a contract to produce such a book was signed with a group of four academics, one of whom was a prominent medical ethicist. The timeline was such that the handbook was to be delivered to AHEC in the next triennium.

The other matter set in train late in 1999 was an overdue revision of ethical guidelines for medical research involving Aboriginal and Torres Strait Islander peoples. The existing guidelines known as the *Guidelines on Ethical Matters in Aboriginal and Torres Strait Islander Health Research* (Interim Guidelines) had been issued by the NHMRC in 1991. They had been controversial from the outset (hence the subtitle

'Interim'), primarily because the people to whom the guidelines were to apply made it clear that they had not been adequately consulted and had no sense of ownership of the document. Despite this past history, the AHEC executive agreed to a process whereby a number of hand-picked Indigenous researchers and health workers were to be invited to form a working party to undertake the revision. While letters of invitation were sent, the working party had not met at the time the 1997–9 triennium ended. As the NHMRC rules state that at the end of a triennium all committees and working parties are disbanded, this left flexibility for the new AHEC to better handle this sensitive issue.

Another surprise invitation

As the end of the triennium neared, AHEC members were asked individually by NHMRC staff (for conveying to the Minister) whether they wished to be considered for reappointment. I was ambivalent as I felt that I had not contributed much and wondered if I had the enthusiasm to be travelling regularly to Canberra. I think that I conveyed my ambivalence to the staff. I was therefore very surprised a couple of months later to receive a phone call from the Federal Health Minister, Dr Michael Woolridge, asking me if I would consider taking on the role of chair of AHEC for the new triennium. After a little thought I agreed. My thoughts were around the fact that the committee was a well-constructed one with untapped potential, the proposed members mentioned by the Minister were very fine people, and that having a non-ethicist as a type of neutral chair might work well. I went in with my eyes open as I was well aware of some of the challenges ahead.

The talent on the new AHEC was quite remarkable. The members included Jesuit priest and ethicist Father Bill Uren, philosopher Dr Christopher Cordner, academic lawyer and ethicist Professor Colin Thomson, philosopher and ethicist Dr Bernadette Tobin and a television journalist with training in health ethics, Ms Belinda Byrne. I knew that my lack of expertise in ethical theory was well-compensated for. Minister Woolridge, aware that one of AHEC's tasks was to revise the *Guidelines on Ethical Matters in Aboriginal and Torres Strait Islander Health Research*, also appointed Mr Robert Griew, a health administrator with extensive experience of working in Indigenous health. His expertise, contacts, and the respect in which he was held in this field proved to be enormously valuable.

The Minister and the NHMRC leave it in the hands of each principal committee of the NHMRC such as AHEC to appoint its own deputy chair. I had been very impressed with the contributions of academic lawyer and ethicist, Professor Colin Thomson, on the previous AHEC and I felt that his background would complement mine. Fortunately, in canvassing each AHEC member, I found that he was by far everybody's first choice. He proved to be an indefatigable contributor and as Deputy Chair a wonderful support to me. Later he also served as Chair of AHEC.

AHEC was resourced by staff of the NHMRC, who were recruited from within the wider staff of the Federal Department of Health. They were uniformly bright, hard-working and dedicated people but were not selected for their capacity to develop from scratch the type of products expected of AHEC. For example, the *National Statement* issued in the previous triennium represented the output of a large working party, the majority of which were AHEC members. Thus if you were appointed to AHEC and were asked to join such a working party, you could expect to do a lot of unpaid work, especially if you volunteered to draft and/or edit documents or sections of documents between meetings of any working party. As the new triennium unfolded, I realised what a slacker I had been during the previous three years.

Revising the guidelines for Indigenous health research

One of the important items on the agenda at the first meeting of the new AHEC was how were we to tackle the task of revising the guidelines for Indigenous health research. My only insight was that AHEC had to find a way in which the new guidelines were to be truly owned by Indigenous Australians but I had absolutely no idea how that might be achieved. The task was made harder by the absence of any Indigenous members on AHEC. Fortunately, Robert Griew spoke up and succinctly outlined a way forward. This involved Robert Griew first travelling across Australia with Aboriginal health researcher, Daniel McAullay, to discuss the revision process with stakeholders and then reporting back to AHEC. This led to a meeting in Melbourne with a broadly representative group of leaders in Indigenous health from across the nation. This group was asked to advise AHEC on what process might best work and what they hoped for from the process.

The rest of this story needs to be told from an Indigenous perspective as I cannot do it justice. What I can say is that AHEC succeeded in engaging successfully with virtually all the key stakeholders, thanks to the work of Robert Griew, Daniel McAullay, Professor Ian Anderson, Shane Houston and others. The end result, an excellent document entitled *Values and Ethics: Guidelines for Ethical Conduct in Aboriginal and Torres Strait Islander Health Research*, was entirely the work of Aboriginal and Torres Strait Islander people. I saw AHEC's task as supporting these people and then shepherding the guidelines through the final approval stage. Although I had no intellectual input into the document, my association with its production gave me great pride.

Throughout the process of developing the guidelines, there was an unresolvable tension between a small group of Aboriginal health workers in NSW and those in the rest of the nation. The sole Aboriginal council member of the NHMRC was affiliated with the NSW group. Having voiced no issues or concerns at Council meetings where progress was regularly reported, he surprised fellow Council members by effectively vetoing the final document when it was presented to a meeting of the full Council for approval. Out of respect for his views, and without fully understanding what the fight was about, the Council decided to defer the decision. The next meeting of Council took place in a new triennium; there were different Aboriginal members present and the new guidelines were enthusiastically approved.

Working with the Law Reform Commission

While in each triennium AHEC starts with an agreed work plan, sometimes new issues emerge whereby Government requests urgent advice. I have already mentioned the request in the previous triennium for a report on the ethics of human cloning. Early in my first triennium as chair (2000–3), we received an urgent request but one with a difference. At the time, the use and misuse of genetic testing, particularly in life insurance but also in employment and other areas, was the subject of controversy and public concern. The Federal Government determined to address those concerns through a detailed inquiry and AHEC was asked to assist the Australian Law Reform Commission (ALRC) in this huge task.

AHEC was in practice the 'junior partner' in this exercise as genetic testing in medical practice and in medical research were only small aspects of the inquiry that was conducted. The President of the ALRC then was Professor David Weisbrot. He made AHEC a very welcome partner and as a result, I felt after the long project was over that AHEC had made a good contribution to the two-volume final report entitled *Essentially Yours: The Protection of Human Genetic Information in Australia.** AHEC also benefited considerably through its involvement. While the NHMRC is obliged to undertake public consultations in producing guidelines, these consultations until this time had been based almost entirely on written submissions, invited after the circulation of draft guidelines. The ALRC also used that approach but

---

*   http://www.alrc.gov.au/publications/essentially-yours-protec-tion-human-genetic-information-australia-alrc-report-96/executi.

supplemented the consultation process through the conduct of public forums across the nation as well as holding meetings with key stakeholders. By observing and participating in the ALRC approach, we learned much that was later applied in a sensitive public consultation on animal to human transplantation research. Through my involvement with ALRC, I got to know David Weisbrot well and we have remained friends (and occasional collaborators) ever since.

Other projects, expected and unexpected

One of the tasks inherited from the previous AHEC eventually arrived on our desks. It was the *Human Research Ethics Handbook.*[†] AHEC was expecting a practical handbook that would help members of human research ethics committees (HRECs) in their task of evaluating health research projects proposed in their institutions. What we received could best be described as an academic treatise on almost every ethical issue that might arise in health and medical research. At consecutive meetings, AHEC discussed what we could do with the document. We were close to deciding to reject the product, accept that we had wasted $40,000 and make a fresh start when Deputy Chairman, Colin Thomson, had another suggestion, accompanied by a generous offer. He advised AHEC that within the long document he had discerned a lot of valuable material and he suggested that with culling, editing and reorganisation, the handbook could be rescued and aligned with the *National Statement* in way that should be useful for HRECs. Furthermore, he offered to undertake this task on an honorary basis. And this Colin did, demonstrating

† https://www.nhmrc.gov.au/guidelines-publications/e42.

his remarkable editing and writing skills. The end result was a presentable product that was issued in 2001. At its launch, Minister Kay Patterson thanked only the original four authors. Colin Thomson's rescue of the document was acknowledged in the introduction to the handbook where his 'skilled editing' was diplomatically referred to.

During my first three years as chair of AHEC, we had no fixed budget and Council seemed prepared to support many of our initiatives. As a follow-up to the release of the *National Statement*, ideas about doing more to support the 200 human research ethics committees (HRECs) in our universities, hospitals and research institutes were tossed around. We ambitiously embarked on four projects, including producing a regular newsletter for HRECs, being prepared to provide speakers at no cost to HREC workshops around the nation, convening a biennial conference for HREC members and providing a 'hot line' for advice about the application of the *National Statement*. In hindsight, this work plan was probably too ambitious and some of it may well have been beyond the statutory remit of AHEC. None of these initiatives survived in the longer term. There were, however, some unanticipated spin-offs.

Research governance issues emerge

Through the increased visibility of AHEC, we began to receive complaints about how some HRECs were going about their work and about their decisions. Most commonly these arose with hospital HRECs. These were not simple matters to deal with, and in some instances the prima facie cases for, at the least, a serious misjudgement, or for decisions involving undeclared conflicts of interest, were of concern to AHEC. We tried as a committee to seek to have each institution address the complaints internally. It was through this approach that it dawned on me that the problems generally were not due to the HREC. Rather it was that most hospitals did not have a clear framework for research governance and that as a result, hospital HRECs were at times obliged to assume an inappropriate role in research governance. Research governance is defined as the 'framework through which institutions are accountable for the scientific quality, ethical acceptability and safety of the research they sponsor'. It therefore encompasses much more than just prospective ethical review of research proposals, which is the focus of HRECs. AHEC then discussed how this could be addressed in the longer term. The method we chose was probably the only one open to us, but in hindsight we chose the wrong target for our message.

AHEC decided that research governance would be the key theme of the second biennial HREC conference. We invited experts on research governance (Dr Terry Stacey from the UK National Health Service and Dr Greg Koski from the USA Office of Research Integrity) to be speakers at the conference. They were both excellent speakers and contributed wholeheartedly to the event. However, when mixing with HREC members during the breaks, I realised that our visitors were speaking to the wrong people. The message about overarching research governance policy needed to be addressed to hospital CEOs and Boards of Management and not to HREC members who had little influence on hospital policy. Despite this mal-direction, some good did come out of the conference.

As the program committee convenor, I was keen that we have a segment where three institutional leaders, from the university sector, a research institute and a major public hospital, spoke on research governance in their sectors. I was aware that the Alfred Hospital in Melbourne had a very active and effective HREC led by Professor John McNeil and a very talented CEO, Dr Michael Walsh, and I thought that Dr Walsh would be the right person to speak about the hospital sector. He accepted the invitation and gave a well-researched and clear presentation. Later we were chatting and he told me that before the invitation arrived he had never given research governance much thought but now that he had done all this research, he had become aware that his hospital needed to do much better in this area. My guess was that this applied to most Australian hospitals at that time.

Over the next few months I urged him to turn his paper into an article for publication but as a busy administrator he never seemed to find the time. I therefore volunteered to write it for him and also drew John McNeill into the task. There was a lot of work and some additional research so that I felt justified in joining them as the third author. The paper was published in the *Medical Journal of Australia** in 2005 and was the first-time research governance had been mentioned in the Australian medical and hospital sectors. The paper identified four key NHMRC documents that form the basis of research governance. They are the *National Statement on Ethical Conduct in Research Involving Humans*; the *Australian*

---

* Walsh, M K, McNeil, J J and Breen, K J, 'Improving the governance of health research', *Medical Journal of Australia*, vol. 182, 2005: 468–71.

Code for the Responsible Conduct of Research; Values and Ethics: Guidelines for Ethical Conduct in Aboriginal and Torres Strait Islander Health Research; and the *Australian Code of Practice for the Care and Use of Animals for Scientific Purposes.* With a little lobbying, research governance also found its way into the hospital accreditation process of the Australian Council on Health Care Standards.

And many other issues

Other things were happening within the NHMRC at this time. As chair of AHEC, I was a member of Council and also a member of its executive committee, along with the chairs of the other three principal committees (the Research Committee, the Health Advisory Committee and the short-lived Strategic Research Development Committee). I had a lot of respect for the chairs of the first two committees. NHMRC had a system whereby each principal committee provided a 'member-in-common' to the other three committees. I accepted the role as member-in-common of the Strategic Research Development Committee (SRDC). At the first meeting I attended, I, along with the member-in-common from the Research Committee, felt obliged to abstain from voting on the first item of business which was to award a large sum of money to an initiative that appeared to us to involve an unresolved conflict of interest. I knew then that I could not stay and soon pleaded workloads as an excuse to be relieved from my role.

During my first term, the NHMRC executive committee was involved in what became known as the 'Bruce Hall affair',* an investigation conducted by the University of New South Wales into allegations of research misconduct. Our role was indirect in that the NHMRC had an interest in seeing that research funds awarded by the Council were utilised appropriately. There is nothing that I learned that is not now on the public record. However, the experience did influence my views on whether universities might better be relieved of investigating their own (see Chapter 11).

During my first three years as chair of AHEC, I had my only appearance before a Senate Committee. I came away very disenchanted. I was there in a support role but was questioned about the work of AHEC in revising its guidelines on in vitro fertilisation – the IVF guidelines (*Ethical guidelines on the use of assisted reproductive technology in clinical practice and research* 2004). This was at a time when human cloning was a hotly debated issue and our Parliament was on its way to passing legislation banning it. I was aware that AHEC's Canadian counterpart had been severely criticised for issuing guidelines that appeared to pre-empt deliberation by the Canadian Parliament on this issue. Because of this background, AHEC had held back its finalisation of its IVF guidelines. I was asked by a member of the Senate in very dismissive language why AHEC had chosen this approach. I replied as courteously and fully as possible but I doubt if the questioner was interested in my reply. My only recollection now is that the meeting took place at about 9.00 pm and that I gained the impression that the behaviour of some of the senators was juvenile in the extreme and possibly influenced by what they had drunk over dinner. The only senator who

* https://www.mja.com.au/system/files/issues/180_04_160204/van 10035_fm.pdf.

142

behaved admirably and with great respect for those called before the committee was the late Senator Brian Harradine.

As a distant outcome of AHEC's report into human cloning, in 2002 the Federal Parliament passed the *Research Involving Human Embryos Act 2002* which established within the framework of the NHMRC, the Embryo Research Licensing Committee. A separate act, the *Prohibition of Human Cloning for Reproduction Act 2002*, banned human cloning. I was asked by the Minister to be AHEC's nominee on this licensing committee from its outset. The committee was very well led by its chair, Professor Jock Findlay, and I became respectful of the difficult task that it was given. I became aware that there was at least one in vitro fertilisation centre that wished to stretch the envelope and was difficult for the committee to deal with. I never felt deeply engaged in the work of the committee and struggled to understand the science involved. After less than twelve months, I sought to be relieved of this role. I am sure that my absence had no impact on the work of the committee.

Animal to human tissue transplantation

Another unscheduled task arose during my first triennium as chair of AHEC. The NHMRC was concerned that research involving transplanting animal tissues or organs into humans (also known scientifically as xenotransplantation) was on the horizon and Australia had no guidelines to adequately protect research subjects. In the process that followed I made some judgements that I came to regret. The issue was first discussed at the NHMRC Executive Committee where I suggested that instead of giving the task to AHEC, it might be wiser to have a more broadly-based group to develop the guidelines. This idea was accepted and the NHMRC assembled a small working party with nominees drawn from AHEC, the NHMRC gene technology advisory committee (this group had done some preliminary work on xenotransplantation) and the NHMRC Animal Welfare Committee. I accepted the task of chairing the working party.

By this time, I had been exposed to the public consultation processes of the Australian Law Reform Commission and as a result, our working party sought to emulate these. We prepared a detailed consultation document and embarked on a consultation process which included a series of community forums as well as the standard receipt of written submissions. Perth was chosen as the site of the first public forum. It was well advertised and we received some media coverage ahead of the event. However, we had made a bad mistake in that, in the afternoon ahead of the public meeting, we agreed to meet separately with a group of interested health consumers assembled by a Perth-based health consumer member of the NHMRC Council. This meeting went well, as expected. What we had not counted on was that by agreeing to this meeting, we had taken away half of the attendees at the evening public meeting. I anticipated trouble when I was informed, and then saw, that animal rights activists were protesting outside the venue for the meeting.

The public meeting was the most difficult meeting I have chaired. The audience consisted almost entirely of people concerned with animal rights. The antipathy in the room to the very notion of animal to human transplantation was almost palpable. Fortunately, there was no violence or threat of violence. The comments and questions to our working party members were however all negative and laced with cynicism and anger. All we could do was to remain calm and polite and make it clear that the views expressed were valuable and respected and would be taken on board.

The central issues in this consultation related to the ethics of using animals in this manner and the risk that viral infections might be transmitted from animals to man. Because of this risk, it was likely that transplant recipients and their close contacts would require long term follow-up. If this were so, then not only would consent for the research be required of the recipient but also consent of close contacts. As a representative working party, its membership included a doctor who was actively researching xenotransplantation. The stakes were high because a number of companies were interested in supporting such research, anticipating a commercial bonanza should a breakthrough occur. In addition to the obstacle of possible viral transmission, it had become clear that any animal species that might be used would need to be genetically modified to overcome the intense immune reaction in human recipients. It became obvious early in our deliberations that the doctor researcher had assumed that the working party was going to produce permissive guidelines. He persisted with this assumption even as the submissions we were receiving were almost all opposed to xenotransplantation research involving humans until the risks of infection were better understood. I wanted to argue very strongly in favour of declaring a moratorium on human research for the time being but, as the chair, I kept my views to myself and let the process run.

The working party produced a second document in the form of draft guidelines for a second round of public consultation and for public meetings held in all capital cities. However, the work was not completed in that triennium and with a new triennium, the opportunity arose to broaden the membership of the working party. I also took the opportunity to ask the NHMRC to find a new chair for the working party so that I could have the freedom to bring my own views to the debate. We were never able to achieve a unanimous view on all the issues and so we ended up taking to the Council a document that provided very strict guidelines should Council give the go-ahead for human research. As I partly anticipated, Council members observed that the guidelines were so strict that they were unlikely to be met, indicating that in the present state of knowledge, it was probably too risky to proceed. Council therefore rejected the guidelines and instead announced a five year moratorium on involving humans in any research. Animal to animal transplantation research could continue.

That was the end of my involvement in the debates around xenotransplantation although I have closely followed subsequent developments. Towards the end of the five-year moratorium, the NHMRC, now led by a new Chief Executive Officer, commenced a process of reviewing the need for the moratorium. The outcome was a foregone conclusion as the review was conducted by an expert scientific panel rather than by a broad-based working party including persons representing the community and other stakeholders. The panel recommended that the moratorium be lifted. This recommendation was accepted by Council but then the Council referred the matter back to AHEC with a request that AHEC now produce ethical guidelines that would need to be met for any institutional HREC to approve such human research. The new draft guidelines seemed to me to be similar to the document that the NHMRC working party had produced ten years earlier. My sense of the draft guidelines was that any human research ethics committee asked to consider an animal to human research proposal would find it difficult to be reassured about the overall safety of such research in the present state of scientific knowledge. On the other hand, I am not sure that the decision to proceed with research that carries a risk for the entire community (through possible spread of a new viral disease) rather than a risk just to one human subject should be left in the hands of only one of Australia's two hundred human research ethics committees.

Retained human body parts

Another unscheduled task that was referred to AHEC arose from events in the UK that came to light in 1999 known as the Alder Hey Children's Hospital scandal.* The UK public was deeply alarmed to be told that the hospital was illegally retaining parts of human bodies removed at operations or autopsies. Understandably, the media here soon discovered that this was a common practice also in in Australia, although with a significant difference, in that retention of body parts was not illegal and furthermore did not at that time require consent from family members. As a result of this practice, there were large numbers of body parts retained in teaching hospitals across the country. For many family members this

* https://en.wikipedia.org/wiki/Alder_Hey_organs_scandal.

news was distressing. Hospital authorities were in need of advice and guidance as to what to do with their collections. Health Minister Dr Michael Woolridge in November 2000 asked AHEC to take on the task of developing such advice. AHEC member, Dr Christopher Cordner, agreed to chair a working party of key stakeholders and the task was completed promptly. His group's report entitled *Organs Retained at Autopsy – Ethical and Practical Issues*[*] became the basis of nation-wide action in this sensitive area. The guidelines were later replaced by the Australian Health Minister's Advisory Council document *The National Code of Ethical Autopsy Practice.*

Complementary medicines

A task related to my position as Chair of AHEC that I undertook in 2003 was to serve on an Expert Committee on Complementary Medicines in the Health System which was established by the Federal Government Therapeutic Goods Administration (TGA) as one of the government's responses to the recall of over 1,600 complementary medicines manufactured by Pan Pharmaceuticals.[†] Its task was massive as it was asked to 'consider the regulatory, health system and industry structures necessary to ensure that the central objectives of the National Medicines Policy are met in relation to complementary medicines.' The committee was large and was divided on almost every issue by the vastly different philosophies of the members whose background was in orthodox medicine and those who worked in

* https://www.nhmrc.gov.au/guidelines-publications/e41.
† https://www.tga.gov.au/expert-committee-complementary-medi-cines-health-system.

manufacturing or dispensing complementary medicines. Its secretariat was provided by the section of TGA responsible for the oversight of complementary medicines.

Membership of the Expert Committee included a naturopath. At the first meeting, there was some discussion about the need for evidence of efficacy and the use of clinical trials. The naturopath defended the general absence of clinical trials in his field by explaining that clinical trials would undermine the 'mystique' of naturopathic remedies. I struggled to really engage in the work of the committee. I felt that the secretariat was determined that our final report would not put a huge industry at risk. There was clearly no possibility that the 'registration' of complementary medicines in Australia was ever going to be subject to the evidence required of orthodox medicines. Thus to this day, the general public wrongly assumes that because a complementary medicine product has been approved for sale by the TGA, the product has been proven to be safe and to do what it claims to do.

As my appointment to the Committee was described as providing expertise in 'ethical issues associated with the promotion and use of medicines', I wrote a short treatise for the committee on what I felt were the key ethical issues surrounding the use of complementary medicines. My input had no impact on the final report although, to his great credit, the chair of the working party did insert a strong ethical tone to the report through his 'Chairman's preface'. I later was invited by a fellow committee member to edit my treatise for publication and this I did.‡ In that

‡ Breen, K J, 'Ethical issues in the use of complementary medicines', *Climacteric*, 6, 2003: 268–72.

paper, I argued that the Australian regulatory system for medicines could be said to be 'designed to minimize and conceal the differences between scientifically proven medicines and those which are unproven, thereby deceiving the community'. I do not expect the system to be changed by government as the complementary and alternative medicine industry is seen as an economic benefit to the nation.

Another three years of work

As we neared the next triennium, I had some ideas about the ownership of the *National Statement* that I would pursue if reappointed. While I have implied criticism of my predecessor's approach to having the *National Statement* endorsed by a number of relevant national organisations so late in its development, I nevertheless felt that the idea had great merit. It was the timing and lack of consultation with stakeholders that was the problem. In this new triennium, two key NHMRC documents were due for revision. One was the *National Statement* and the other was the *Australian Code for the Responsible Conduct of Research* (formerly known as the *Joint NHMRC/AVCC Statement and Guidelines on Research Practice*). Through the NHMRC executive committee, I proposed that it would be in the nation's interests if the two documents could be seen to be complementary, and owned and issued jointly by three key stakeholders, viz. the NHMRC, the Australian Research Council and Universities Australia. Fortunately, this idea was acted upon and soon agreement was reached that this would happen. As a result, the 2007 edition of the *National Statement* and the 2007 *Australian Code for the Responsible Conduct of Research* were developed by joint working parties of the NHMRC, Australian Research Council and Universities Australia. The working party revising the *National Statement* was chaired by AHEC member, Dr Christopher Cordner, while the *Code of Responsible Conduct* working party was chaired by Professor Warwick Anderson, who had recently completed six years as chair of the research committee of the NHMRC and who later was appointed CEO of the NHMRC. I served on both working parties and was effectively a member-in-common. I saw my role as seeking to ensure the complementarity of the two documents.

My second triennium as chair of AHEC (2004–6) promised to be just as busy as my first but having over-extended myself in the previous triennium, I sought now to avoid being too personally involved in some of AHEC's projects. The projects included a revision of the *National Statement*, the development of guidelines for the care of patients in the vegetative state, the production of a guide for Aboriginal and Torres Strait Islander peoples to assist them in applying the *Values and Ethics* document, and the convening of a second national conference for members of human research ethics committees. Fortunately, the new Health Minister, Ms Kay Patterson, gave us a strong committee. Although Dr Bernadette Tobin did not seek reappointment, there was considerable continuity of membership from the previous AHEC as well as some new talent. The new talent included Darwin-based Indigenous Australian, Ms Terry Dunbar, with whose capacities I had become familiar with through her membership of the working party that developed the

Values and Ethics guidelines. AHEC had requested that we have two Indigenous Australians on the committee but despite Minister Patterson's best intentions, this did not happen, so Terry Dunbar was on her own.

Terry Dunbar proved to be a superb contributor to the work of AHEC. She led a working party that undertook a wide consultation with Indigenous Australians and with research ethics committees that were frequently involved in assessing research proposals involving Indigenous Australians. Her team produced a valuable and practical document entitled *Keeping research on track: A guide for ATSI peoples about health research ethics*. This was warmly supported and approved by AHEC and the NHMRC.

Other matters referred to AHEC in my second triennium as chair included a request that NHMRC guidelines on informed consent be revised and a request that AHEC examine the question of whether quality assurance studies in health care represented research and hence required prospective review by a human research ethics committee. With regard to the former, we advised the Council that the informed consent guidelines did not warrant revision but instead, a complementary guideline on good communication would be a useful addition. Out of this came the NHMRC document entitled *Communicating with Patients. Advice for Medical Practitioners*. With regard to the latter, a working party that included AHEC members and external community members chaired by AHEC deputy chair, Dr Bryan Campbell, produced a practical short document entitled *When Does Quality Assurance in Health Care Require Independent Ethical Review*. The document took the approach that prior ethical review of quality assurance work should rarely be required. I was happy with this outcome as I had sensed that we might be accused of 'ethics creep' should we take the opposite view. 'Ethics creep' is a term used in a critical or derogatory sense to imply that ethics committees are seeking to insert themselves into more and more areas of human activity, resulting in unnecessary and inefficient ethical oversight.

Working with Health Ministers

I have mentioned earlier my mostly satisfactory interactions with three Victorian health ministers and have given some insights into the good work of Dr Michael Woolridge as a federal health minister, both in relation to AHEC and to the Australian Medical Council. In my second three-year stint as chair of AHEC, the relevant minister at the start was Ms Kay Patterson. She appointed a very impressive array of new and old faces for AHEC for the new triennium. She was responsive to a request from the NHMRC that AHEC have two Aboriginal members for this term. Ms Terry Dunbar from Darwin had accepted one of the positions and Minister Patterson had approached an experienced and highly respected Aboriginal health advocate from Western Australia. At the last minute, he was unable to take up the appointment and AHEC met on a couple of occasions lacking one member.

In the interim, Prime Minister Howard undertook a ministerial reshuffle resulting in Mr Tony Abbott taking over as Health Minister. Ignoring the NHMRC request for a second Aboriginal member, he filled the AHEC vacancy with a bioethicist, Dr Nick Tonti-Filippini, who by now was well-recognised as holding conservative Catholic views on most ethical issues. On hearing this news, I sensed immediately that the role of the chair of AHEC was going to be a lot more stressful in this triennium. My prediction came true at the first meeting Dr Tonti-Filippini attended.

At this meeting an important agenda item was the final sign off of revised guidelines for IVF (*Ethical guidelines on the use of assisted reproductive technology in clinical practice and research 2004*). The guidelines had been developed over a period of nearly three years and two rounds of public consultation by a broadly representative working party chaired by AHEC member, Dr Bernadette Tobin. Recognising that contentious IVF issues including preimplantation genetic testing, sex selection, and surrogacy were really matters for Parliament rather than AHEC, the working party recommended that these simply be briefly noted in the document but not otherwise formally addressed. AHEC had debated earlier drafts of the guidelines and was confident, through its extensive consultations, that they would be welcomed by the vast majority of practitioners in this clinical field. Dr Tonti-Filippini argued vigorously that the guidelines were incomplete in that they lacked a definition of a human embryo. Committee members were clearly unsure of what Tonti-Filippini was after. I wondered about his motives and what he was seeking to achieve.

I decided to use the chair's authority by explaining that after two rounds of public consultation on drafts that did not contain a definition of an embryo, his request was outside the legislated framework for consultation, and the related duty to take heed of any submissions, and that such an amendment could not be added at this late stage. AHEC supported my view and the document was approved unchanged. To accommodate Dr Tonti-Filippini, I suggested that AHEC could refer his request for a definition of a human embryo to the next meeting of the NHMRC. I had in mind that I would advise Council that, if the task was accepted, it should be allocated to the Embryo Research Licensing Committee, and not to AHEC, and this is indeed what happened.*

Another hiccup occurred soon after this. Over a coffee break, Dr Tonti-Filippini confided in me that he had been advised by Minister Abbott that his appointment was intended as a means of 'keeping an eye' on the work of AHEC. I tried to confirm this statement by speaking with a senior advisor to the Minister who denied this was the intention. For the rest of the triennium, I was anticipating difficulties with this AHEC member but apart from attitudes that seemed to not endear him to some of the women members of AHEC, the time passed uneventfully. To Dr Tonti-Filippini's credit, I was reliably informed that in the following triennium, he did an excellent job chairing an AHEC working party that finalised the development of new guidelines for care of people in an unresponsive or minimally responsive state.†

My next dealing with Minister Abbott was to invite him to speak at our forthcoming second conference for human research ethics committee members in Canberra. He was

---

* *'Human Embryo' – A Biological Definition.* https://www.nhmrc. gov.au/_files_nhmrc/file/research/embryos/reports/humanem-bryo.pdf.
† *Ethical guidelines for the care of people in post-coma unresponsiveness.* https://www.nhmrc.gov.au/_files_nhmrc/publications/attach-ments/e81.pdf.

keen to accept the invitation, went to the trouble to speak with me briefly about what themes might be appropriate to this audience, and requested that I send his office a selection of recent publications relevant to the work of human research ethics committees and to the work of AHEC. We were expecting an interesting talk. His attendance attracted several journalists. I was dismayed when he chose to speak on the topic of third trimester abortions in Melbourne public hospitals. This was not relevant to the work of human research ethics committees and in my view was chosen simply to use the opportunity to lecture the captive journalists in attendance about his personal views. I was not impressed.

My third and last dealing with him was about a year before my second term as chair was to end. He asked to see me about a project that he had in mind for AHEC. Accompanied by our most senior member of AHEC's secretariat, I attended on him in his office at Parliament House. His request was for AHEC to commission research into a series of 'clinical cases raising ethical issues' that ethics committees were handling in hospitals across Australia. Knowing that this was in fact a directive, we simply accepted the task. I knew that there was little point in explaining that human research ethics committees dealt with research and not with clinical care (apart from a small number of hospitals that had chosen for pragmatic reasons to combine their clinical ethics committee with the research ethics committee).

I suspected that his project was planned to be a backdoor means of the Minister finding ethical decisions which conflicted with his personal philosophy. I was aware that such a project, needing to be put out to tender and then followed by a considerable amount of work, would probably take a couple of years to complete and that when it was completed, it was likely that neither Minister Abbott nor I would be involved with AHEC. There were some very good proposals made when tenders were called for. A small academic group based in Melbourne was awarded the task. They did an excellent job and their report published in December 2006 was a fine testament to the work done by Australia's volunteer members of human research ethics committees.* By this date, I was no longer a member of AHEC, but Mr Abbott was still the Minister for Health. The report focussed on ethical issues in human research.

This is as good a place as any to tell an oft repeated tale about the workings of HRECs. Members would frequently amuse each other by recounting stories of bioethicists being appointed to HRECs and being observed by colleagues as unable to make a decision on any of the research protocols being considered by the committees. While apocryphal, these stories probably contain an element of truth. Fortunately, the *National Statement*, while advising on several core categories of members for HRECs, does not deem bioethicists to be required members.

Ethical standards in medical practice and medical research have evolved to be pretty much universal, although cultural, economic, political and developmental influences exist at the local level. Through my role with AHEC, I had the privilege of observing, and at times participating in, international activities designed to share ideas around ethical issues in health care and in medical research. Through these meetings, my appreciation of the structure and composition of AHEC

* *Challenging Ethical Issues in Contemporary Research on Human Beings* https://www.nhmrc.gov.au/guidelines-publications/e73.

was greatly increased for I found that the equivalent bodies, often called national bioethics committees or commissions, had very different compositions, most often being composed entirely of specialist bioethicists. By comparison, AHEC's composition, prescribed in the *NHMRC* Act, guarantees that a much broader range of views, hopefully approximating those of the Australian public, are brought to bear on contentious matters.

Challenges ahead for AHEC

Whether AHEC is referred such contentious issues to consider has become less certain under amendments to the *NHMRC* Act made in 2006. These amendments changed the reporting relationship of AHEC. Previously AHEC reported to and through the full Council of the NHMRC. Under the changes to the Act, not only does AHEC now report and respond to the Chief Executive Officer but so too does the Council and its President. This changed reporting relationship is emphasised in the following introduction to AHEC that now appears on the NHMRC website: 'One of the CEO's functions under the NHMRC Act is to inquire into, issue guidelines on, and advise the community on ethical issues relating to health. This function includes the issuing of human research guidelines.' In addition, the legislation now states that before the Health Minister can refer a matter to AHEC, there must be consultation with the CEO of the NHMRC. This requirement seems at odds with the desirable independence of AHEC and may limit its opportunities to contribute to debates over contentious ethical issues in health. As noted earlier in this chapter, under the then legislation, referrals from the Health Minister of the day included the fraught issues of human cloning, genetic testing and stored human remains. One has to ask why should the CEO's approval now be required for such referrals?

My impression is that these changes in reporting relationships have had an adverse effect on the range and nature of the tasks given to AHEC, its capacity to influence debate and discussion of important ethical issues around health care and health care research, and on its visibility to the public. How much of this change is unintended or perhaps even due to budget restraints is unclear. One very noticeable change has been the cessation of the biannual continuing education conference for members of Australia's 200 human research ethics committees.

Until amendments to the *NHMRC* Act were made in 2006, the membership of AHEC was to a large degree protected from political influence and manipulation in two ways. The Federal Minister for Health was obliged to seek nominations for several categories of membership from relevant peak national organisations. For the positions of chair of AHEC, and the member with expertise in medical ethics, the Minister was obliged to consult with the eight state and territory health ministers. These requirements, which reduced the possibility of politically motivated appointments, were removed with the 2006 amendments.[*] These changes worried me at the time but to date no Minister for Health seems to have done anything other than seek to achieve a talented and balanced AHEC membership.

* For a discussion of the 2006 amendments see Chapter 8 Human Research Ethics Guidelines in Australia in *Big Picture Bioethics: Developing Democratic Policy in Contested Domains*. Edited by Dodds S and Ankeny R A. Springer, 2016.

Chapter 10

GOOD MEDICAL PRACTICE AND PROFESSIONALISM

Updating our textbook

As our 1997 textbook *Ethics Law and Medical Practice* was well-received, we always planned to produce a new edition. Finding the time to do this proved difficult until I decided in 2006 that it was time for me to give up my sessional appointment at St Vincent's Public Hospital in Melbourne. I had been on the senior medical staff since 1972, initially in a full-time appointment, but reduced to a sessional appointment in 1997 when I returned from long service leave. While it was no longer compulsory to retire from the hospital at the age of sixty-five, I felt that I should do so since it would free up a position for a younger physician. I also felt a sense of moral obligation to do this as from the time of my first appointment, I was aware that sixty-five was then the official retiring age. I found that my views placed me in a minority as many of my colleagues were keen to stay on. Some sessional appointees seemed to feel that if they left the hospital, they might be forgotten and their private practice referrals would diminish. I had an additional reason for retiring in that I was no longer enthusiastic nor fully confident about one task that my appointment entailed, viz. the requirement to be on twenty-four-hour call to undertake urgent endoscopic procedures in patients with life-threatening gastrointestinal bleeding.

In leaving the public hospital, I was still going to maintain my private practice as a gastroenterologist. At that time, I was sharing our practice office in Fitzroy with two wonderfully supportive women colleagues. We covered for each other when anyone was away for holidays, conferences and the like. Through my NHMRC commitments, I was away far more often than my colleagues. I saw myself as entering a phase of partial retirement from clinical practice but this was not to be. In seeking to work part-time as a gastroenterologist, I had not counted on several factors that would weigh on my mind. First, patients with diseases of the gut and the liver do not have part-time illnesses and I found that I felt guilty if I was not available to them. Referring family doctors likewise prefer you to be around full-time. While my two colleagues would still cover for me as needed, I was very reluctant to request this help when my reason for being unavailable was to be out playing golf! I soon made the decision that I would give up my plan to do part-time clinical work and instead would retire from all clinical work. This I did at the end of 2008. My decision was made easier by now having a part-time appointment as a member of the Federal Administrative Appeals Tribunal. This provided well-paid intellectually stimulating work, and combined with the task of revising our textbook, I was confident that through these roles, I would not miss clinical practice. And so it proved to be.

Vernon Plueckhahn was no longer able to be deeply involved in the new edition of our book but fortunately Stephen Cordner was. Recalling that our 1997 edition was criticised by one reviewer for not having a legally qualified co-author, Stephen and I agreed to recruit such a person. Colin Thomson, ACT based academic lawyer with a strong interest in medical ethics, who I first met when we were members of the Australian Health Ethics Committee from 1997–2000, was the obvious choice. As described earlier in this book, Colin has excellent writing skills and his expertise and knowledge base complemented ours. Luckily, he was very willing to be involved.

Finding a new publisher

We soon found that our publisher, Allen and Unwin, was not as keen as we were with the idea of a new edition. It seemed that the company felt that its brief experiment with this type of book should not continue. As all printed copies of the 1997 book had been sold, the company was happy to return copyright to us. Now all we had to do was to find a new publisher. This is not an easy task although it helps if one already has a book that has been published. I made a submission on our behalf to Cambridge University Press, chosen because their Australian office is in Melbourne, and because their catalogue seemed to lack this category of text book. I was pleasantly surprised to be offered an interview with one of their senior publishers, Ms Debbie Lee. The interview went well, greatly helped by the fact that early in our discussions, I became aware that I knew her late father, Dr Julian Lee, who was a well-liked and respected respiratory physician at Royal Prince Alfred Hospital when I was training there in 1969 and 1970. The outcome was that Cambridge University Press took us on. Debbie Lee supported the project wholeheartedly. We were aware that our book needed a more accurate title and struggled to find one until Debbie suggested *Good Medical Practice: Professionalism, Ethics and Law*. We accepted her suggestion immediately.

Good Medical Practice was first used as the title to a valuable document created by the UK General Medical Council* and the title has since been borrowed for an equivalent Australian document, created in 2008 through a joint initiative of the Australian Medical Council and the state and territory medical boards. The Australian document is called *Good medical practice: a code of conduct for doctors in Australia*. It was adopted by the newly formed Medical Board of Australia in 2010. Its purpose is to make explicit the standards of ethical and professional conduct expected of all doctors in Australia. The code also helps doctors understand their responsibilities, is used by the Medical Board as a set of standards of medical practice against which a doctor's professional conduct is assessed and can be used as an educational resource in many settings. I believe that the Australian version is a better structured and more complete guide for doctors than the UK version but this might be a biased opinion as I was a member of the working party that developed the code of conduct. We referred to the

---

* http://www.gmc-uk.org/guidance/good_medical_practice.asp.

GMC Good Medical Practice document in our 2010 edition of our book and were happy to borrow the name, with the additional words 'professionalism, ethics and law' as the title for our third edition. Ethics and law are self-explanatory but 'medical professionalism' deserves a little explication.

Thoughts on medical professionalism

When I first heard mention of 'medical professionalism' nearly two decades ago, my initial reaction was to regard it as a tautology on the basis that medicine is a profession. Since first used by Wynia and colleagues in the *New England Journal of Medicine* in 1999,[*] it has become a popular expression. The term gained more attention in 2002 when a self-appointed group of doctors in North America and Europe promoted a 'charter of medical professionalism'.[†] This was followed in 2005 with a similar document issued by the UK Royal College of Physicians. I did not then[‡] and still do not believe that these documents were particularly relevant to Australia for the following reasons.

First, all three documents claimed that the medical profession was under attack. This may have been true for some doctors in some health care systems in other countries but has never applied in Australia. Second, the authors of the 'charter of medical professionalism' sought to depict

---

[*] Wynia, M K, Latham, S R, Kao, A C et al., 'Medical professionalism in society', *N Eng J Med*, 1999, 341: 1612–16.

[†] 'Medical professionalism in the new millennium: a physicians' charter', *Lancet*, 2002, 359: 520–2.

[‡] See Breen, K, 'Commentary on the physicians' charter', *Lancet*, vol. 359, 2002, p. 2042 and Breen, K J, 'Medical professionalism project', *Medical Journal of Australia*, vol. 178, 2003: 93.

their document as a social contract yet had not bothered to consult the communities with whom the contract was being made. Third, none of the three documents examined in depth other factors at work such as changes in medical practice and health care delivery and increasing pressure on health care budgets in developed nations. Also ignored were past expressions of similar concerns in 1975, 1980 and 1987.

The Australian medical education and health care environments are different from those of the countries in which arose the new emphasis on medical professionalism. These differences include: the teaching of professional attitudes in Australian medical schools under the heading of 'personal and professional development' (this has long been a requirement for accreditation of medical schools by the Australian Medical Council); a health care system that, despite some faults, generally remains equitable and accessible; and a well-developed health consumer movement that ensures patient input into almost every aspect of health care education and health care provision. Despite these differences, most Australian medical colleges have somewhat thoughtlessly embraced this new medical professionalism movement. Fortunately, it is unlikely that any harm will result, while some good may follow, as the teaching of professional attitudes and conduct needs to be reinforced during postgraduate training and to remain built-in to ongoing standards of practice. The extension of Australian Medical Council accreditation of medical schools to the Australian medical colleges (see Chapter 8) was already helping this to happen.

From my perspective, the 2010 edition of our textbook contained what was essentially a complete curriculum for medical professionalism. I was surprised and disappointed that one reviewer was critical of the new edition for not emphasising the 'new' medical professionalism; I guess the 'wood for the trees' metaphor might apply. I made a mental note that our next edition would not be open to this criticism.

An unexpected flow-on

There was an unexpected flow-on from our publishing link with Debbie Lee at Cambridge University Press. A year after the 2010 edition of Good Medical Practice was published I received a phone call from her. She had left Cambridge University Press and was now in charge of publishing at the Australian Council for Educational Research (ACER). There she had observed that ACER held the contracts for designing and delivering the entry examinations, the Graduate Medical School Admissions Test (GAMSAT) and the Undergraduate Medicine and Health Sciences Admission Test (UMAT),* used by nearly all Australian medical schools. She was looking for an author for a new book to guide prospective medical students with the title of 'So You Want to be a Doctor' and she was contacting me to ask if I might be interested in the task. My initial (silent) reaction was to wonder why anyone would need such a book as I certainly did not need one fifty years ago. However, after a few days of reading and thinking, I saw that such a book might help a lot of young people so I accepted Debbie's invitation.

In writing the book, I became very aware of the challenges now facing new entrants to the medical profession. Candidates have to rank well in either the UMAT or

* https://gamsat.acer.org/ and https://umat.acer.edu.au/.

GAMSAT exam, then score well at interview and, for some medical schools, submit a personal portfolio that is also scored. Incidentally, there is no evidence that any of these methods of assessment result in the selection of the people most suited to clinical practice. After a university course of four, five or six years' duration, graduates will emerge with a large debt based on HECS fees or, for some, based on having borrowed money to pay for a place in a medical school.

Early in my research for the new book, I read an informative paper written by Israeli physician, Dr Jochanan Benbassat, and a colleague. They had thoroughly examined all the research surrounding admission processes for medical schools and had concluded that the only reliable measure was prior academic achievement which predicted completion of the medical course and nothing more. They recommended that the medical school entry process should instead focus on ensuring that students are well-informed as to what lies ahead in the medical course and after graduation. I chose this perceptive advice as the theme of my book, which was published in 2012 with the full title of *So You Want to Be a Doctor: A guide for prospective medical students in Australia*. I entered into email correspondence with Dr Benbassat and he generously agreed to join a small advisory group that would critique drafts of the book. His comments were always the first to arrive. To thank him, I visited Jerusalem to meet him and we have kept in touch since. He has had a long experience in medical education and had an excellent book published by Springer in 2015 entitled *Teaching Professional Attitudes and Basic Clinical Skills to Medical Students: A Practical Guide*. I recommend it to any doctor who supervises or teaches medical students.

167

Debbie Lee subsequently commissioned three other *So You Want to Be* books about becoming teachers, lawyers and veterinary surgeons. I was able to recommend to her Professor David Weisbrot for the book about studying law and another friend, Dr Eric Allan, a vet and a published author, to write about entering his profession. I liked all three books and thought they were all better than mine, with the one on teaching being my first pick.

On keeping a text book up to date

For anyone who has not been involved in keeping a text book up to date, it might be of interest to know how I went about the task for *Good Medical Practice: Professionalism, Ethics and Law* after 2010. There were two phases to the work. From the date of publication, I kept a close watch on approximately ten medical journals and two medical newspapers that regularly carried relevant material. Any material that was likely to be of use was photocopied and filed according to which chapter from the previous edition of our book seemed most relevant. When the revision process began in earnest in 2014, for each chapter under review, a key word literature search was conducted. At the completion of the revision, over half of the 1,100 references in the book were new. We saw the need to add three new chapters. Two of these were introductory in nature and were focussed on defining what good medical practice is and what professionalism means, for we were determined that future readers would be in no doubt that the book fully addressed all the elements of medical professionalism. The third new chapter was on conflicts of interest and doctors' relationships with industry, a theme that had previously formed a small part of a chapter entitled Prescribing and Administering Drugs.

Once again we needed to find a new publisher as Cambridge University Press was no longer keen to be involved. In a way, we were satisfied with their decision because while the company had effective means of promoting its books to university students, it seemed to us that the company lacked experience or methods for promoting our book to the medical profession. In 1997, before we signed with Allen and Unwin, we had explored working with Blackwell and the Australian Medical Council as the two organisations had recently jointly published a textbook for overseas trained doctors. Recalling this, we decided to offer our 2016 (fourth) edition to the Australian Medical Council. Fortunately, the CEO of the Council, Mr Ian Frank, and his team were enthusiastic about the idea.

The Council by this time had become experienced in this type of publishing and was very willing to add our book to their catalogue. As part of the arrangement, we decided to donate all rights to the book to the Council, forgoing all royalties. There were a number of reasons for this decision. We were very conscious that over 100 experts in various fields had helped us to write the four editions of the book and yet there was no easy means of rewarding them for their contributions. All they received each time was a copy of our book and acknowledgement in the book. We had never seen the writing of the book as a means of enriching ourselves. The small royalties earned in the past had been donated to the Victorian Institute of Forensic Medicine for educational purposes. As I had retired from all medical practice, I felt increasingly at risk of becoming out of touch with developments in the many subjects covered in the book. Thus a new edition would need at least one new author and the Council was in a good position to find such a person and to take full responsibility for the book. To the present three authors, this was a satisfying way of planning for the future.

Chapter 11

MISCONDUCT IN MEDICAL RESEARCH

A harm that needs greater recognition

While most people are probably aware of common types of professional misconduct of which doctors are accused, such awareness seems not to extend to misconduct in medical research. This lack of awareness is unfortunate as the harm that can arise from research misconduct, especially poorly conducted research or fabricated research, can extend to many more people than can most categories of professional misconduct engaged in by doctors. One relatively recent example should make this clear. In 1998, Dr Andrew Wakefield, then a respected UK paediatrician, published a research paper in the prestigious medical journal, the *Lancet*. The paper's title was 'Ileal-lymphoid-nodular hyperplasia, non-specific colitis, and pervasive developmental disorder in children',[*] a title that does not hint at its real message which was to link childhood autism to the administration of the measles, mumps and rubella (MMR) vaccine. That message soon became widely disseminated and vaccination rates fell in many countries. In parallel, the incidence of measles and mumps rose, and serious illness and deaths resulted.

* https://en.wikipedia.org/wiki/Andrew_Wakefield.

171

Wakefield's research findings could not be reproduced by several other groups of medical researchers but these negative findings did not restore public confidence in the MMR vaccine. The discovery that Wakefield had falsified findings, that much of the research was conducted unethically, and that he had a major undeclared financial conflict of interest only gradually came to light from 2004 onwards. Actions to address his misconduct and correct the research record did not take place until 2010. In that year he was stripped of his medical registration by the UK General Medical Council and the *Lancet* announced that the 1998 paper was 'retracted'. Retraction is the process used by scientific journals when informed of fraud or of other reasons for serious doubt about the authenticity of a piece of research. It takes the form of an announcement in a later edition of the journal. Often the process is delayed and in the meanwhile the original research paper may have been widely quoted in other journals. The original work remains in printed copies of the journal sitting in libraries around the world. There exists a very informative web site dedicated to keeping track of research that is retracted.*

Since then further work by an investigative journalist has indicated that Wakefield's 'research' was an elaborate fraud and that he had been motivated by a plan to profit from a vaccine scare. Disgraced in the UK, Wakefield has made a new life for himself in the USA where, despite the overwhelming contrary evidence, he continues to deny his misconduct. He has become an international beacon for a small but active percent of the population who are opposed to all forms of vaccination. While this chapter was being written, a local

* For a sense of how frequently research papers are retracted, go to http://retractionwatch.com/.

reverberation of Wakefield's damaging impact gained media attention as a Melbourne general practitioner who is alleged to have supported anti-vaccination groups had his medical registration suspended pending a disciplinary inquiry. Even today, in many countries, vaccination rates 'post-Wakefield' have not recovered to their past good levels. In response, some jurisdictions have resorted to forms of compulsion such as insisting on documented vaccination before enrolment at school to achieve what is termed herd immunity. Wakefield's blatant research fraud and gross misconduct has caused great harm.

How research misconduct is dealt with

My interest in research misconduct was stimulated years ago through reading in the *British Medical Journal* of frequent disciplinary hearings by the General Medical Council into allegations of research misconduct. This frequency seemed discrepant in two ways. First, the GMC seemed to hold fewer inquiries into the other types of misconduct that doctors faced in Australia. Second, research misconduct by doctors seemed to rarely come to the attention of medical boards in the USA or Australia.[†] I later discovered that the first discrepancy was because action by the GMC was forced by an independent investigator[‡] but even today I remain unsure about the second.

[†] Exceptions to this include the case of Dr William McBride in NSW (see https://en.wikipedia.org/wiki/William_McBride_(doctor).

[‡] As discussed in Ch. 11, the General Medical Council was obliged to hold disciplinary hearings when provided with damning evidence of misconduct by doctors received from an investigator employed by the Association of the British Pharmaceutical Industry.

I sought to stimulate the interest of medical boards abroad and in Australia in these issues, without any obvious impact. When I was invited to speak at the International Association of Medical Regulatory Authorities in Canada in 2002, I chose this subject as my theme, using the title 'Research misconduct and the role for regulators'. I later turned that talk into a paper which was published in Australia in the *Internal Medicine Journal*.* The lack of disciplinary action by most medical boards might be explained by the absence of direct 'victims' of research misconduct and that medical board processes generally are activated by a person lodging a complaint. Without somebody who recognises that they have been harmed, and hence might lodge a complaint, it is unlikely that allegations of research misconduct will reach a medical board. As I will discuss below, research misconduct is typically handled within the institution where the research was conducted (universities, research institutes and hospitals mainly); unless the misconduct is thought to be egregious, it is not in the interests of these organisations to notify a medical board of cases of proven misconduct.

It is also possible that institutions do not regard research misconduct by doctors as a form of professional misconduct. This seems regrettable as in searching for deterrents against research misconduct, the likelihood of having to appear before a medical board might be a useful addition. It was argued in a Canadian court some time ago that a medical regulator did not have jurisdiction on misconduct allegations that arose from a complaint received from a patient about a prostate cancer research project in which he

* Breen, K J, 'Misconduct in medical research: whose responsibility?', *Internal Medicine Journal*, vol. 33, 2003: 186–19.

was enrolled. The matter went to a Court of Appeal where three judges ruled unanimously that a physician who is in charge of a research group and who develops a research protocol including diagnostic and therapeutic elements is performing a medical act.† I only became aware of this court case through personal contacts made with medical regulators in Canada. Dr Joelle Lescop, who was for a long time the Registrar of the Quebec medical regulatory agency, drew it to my attention.

Definitions of research misconduct

Definitions of research misconduct can be narrow or broad. In the USA, the definition is contained in national legislation and is narrow, being limited to fraud, fabrication or plagiarism. This narrowness was the result of very strong lobbying by the American scientific community. In many other countries, including Australia, a much wider definition is used. Thus included is 'deception in proposing, carrying out or reporting results of research and deliberate, dangerous, or negligent deviations from accepted practice in carrying out research'.‡ Also included in most definitions are serious or repeated breaches of ethical guidelines. As national guidelines usually encompass issues around authorship, supervision of junior researchers etc., the definition allows for more rigorous enforcement of standards of conduct.

---

† Court of Appeal, Quebec, Canada. Decision number 200-09-003042-006, November 2001.
‡ Medical Research Council (UK), *BMJ*, 1998, 316: 1728–9.

Avoidable serious harms

It continues to surprise me that medical researchers involved in incidents where harm has resulted to research participants seem to escape examination by a medical board and possible suspension of medical registration. Three instances immediately come to mind where avoidable serious harms, including deaths, have resulted from medical research and where the problems could be attributed to failure to follow good research practice. There was the death of a healthy volunteer given an inhaled drug in Baltimore where, among several procedural breaches, known lung side effects were overlooked or ignored in designing the study.* Soon after, also in the USA, there was the death of young man in a gene therapy trial when it was alleged that he did not meet the criteria for entering the trial that had been approved by the university ethics review board.†

In the UK in 2006, six healthy paid volunteers were given an experimental drug, TGN 1412, almost simultaneously (i.e. over twenty minutes). This was the first time the new drug had been given to humans. Almost immediately all six people became seriously ill and developed multiple organ failure. The UK regulator (Medicines and Healthcare Products Regulatory Agency) which conducted the initial investigation found no problem with the research protocol, an amazing outcome given that most medical researchers would never plan to give a completely untested new drug to six people at once. This point was not made until a second

* Steinbrook R, 'Protecting research subjects-the crisis at Johns Hopkins', *NEJM*, 2002, 346: 716–20.
† Zallen, D T, 'US gene therapy in crisis', *Trends in Genetics*, vol. 16, 2000: 272–5.

inquiry was conducted. If the research protocol allowed for giving the drug to multiple people at once, then the ethics committee should also be subject to criticism. If that approach was not specified in the protocol, or was ignored, then the research team deserves the opprobrium. It also seems to me that this terrible occurrence may reflect greed on the part of the company developing the drug; if all had gone well, the necessary data about human safety would have been obtained more rapidly, thereby reducing the costs of the research. Somewhere in this sequence, there must have been doctors involved in the planning or the conduct of this research who in my view need to have their conduct examined.[‡]

To my knowledge, no doctor was ever held accountable for the two events in the USA and the one in the UK. In making that comment, I am not suggesting that negligence, research misconduct or other professional misconduct was necessarily involved in any of these cases. But it is alarming that appropriate investigations to exclude this possibility have not been conducted. Such tragedies continue to occur as exemplified in France in 2016[§] where one volunteer died and three others were seriously harmed in a first-in-man study of a new drug for mood disorders. The report of the inquiry into this tragedy has not yet been published. Perhaps this time, the doctors involved will be subject to scrutiny.

Worryingly, research misconduct is both common and increasing.[¶] This should come as no surprise given the

‡ https://en.wikipedia.org/wiki/TGN1412 and also 'Duff's report calls for changes in way drugs are tested', *BMJ*, 2006, 333: 1240.

§ http://www.abc.net.au/news/2016-01-18/man-dies-after-being-left-brain-dead-in-french-drug-trial/7094254.

¶ Breen, K J, 'Research misconduct – time for a rethink?', *Internal Medicine Journal*, 2016, 46: 728–33.

environment in which biomedical research is conducted. There are many forces at work including academic pressures, not only that of 'publish or perish', but also the expectations of our universities that their staff will attract research funding and will go on to commercialise their breakthrough findings.

How is Australia doing?

So, what is Australia doing about this and how does our regulatory model stand up by international comparisons? A short answer to the first question is 'not enough' and to the second, 'about average'. I have been close to some of these matters in the last few years* and from this viewpoint, I see several weaknesses in the Australian system. These include lack of education about ethics and good research practice for many researchers, inappropriate reliance on institutions to investigate and adjudicate allegations of misconduct, relative absence of significant penalties (deterrence) for proven research misconduct, and processes that are claimed to be in conflict with employment contracts, thereby hampering institutional action.

The current *Australian Code for the Responsible Conduct of Research* dates to 2007. The code is comprehensive, generally clear and officially supported by Australia's universities. The code calls for institutions to ensure that staff are educated about research ethics and good research practice.† My sense

* As mentioned in Ch. 9, I was part of the working party that developed the *Australian Code for the Responsible Conduct of Research* and since 2011 have been a member of the Australian Research Integrity Committee.
† The full wording is 'that institutions provide induction, formal

is that universities seek to comply with this requirement but I am less confident that our major hospitals, where much medical research is conducted, match this effort. It may be that the hospitals do try but that young medical graduates starting out in medical research choose not to engage in educational sessions. There is some support for my sense of this failing from the findings of a study in 2008 that revealed that the group of Australian researchers most lacking in knowledge and awareness of the national guidelines were those who were medically qualified.[‡] The implications of this finding are of concern. If those who supervise new medical researchers are unfamiliar with the guidelines, then what chance do new researchers have?

The *Australian Code for the Responsible Conduct of Research* is divided into two parts. Part A consists of the guidelines and Part B advises institutions about how complaints and allegations of research misconduct are to be handled. In Australia, as in many countries, dealing with allegations of misconduct is the responsibility of the researcher's employing institution, with a proviso that more serious allegations should be evaluated and determined by a panel assembled that is independent of the institution. It is difficult to evaluate how effective the provisions of Part B have been. There are no publicly available data on how many investigations are

---

training and continuing education for all research staff, including research trainees. Training should cover research methods, ethics, confidentiality, data storage and records retention, as well as regulation and governance. Training should also cover the institution's policies regarding responsible research conduct, all aspects of this Code, and other sources of guidance that are available'.

‡ Babl, F E, Sharwood, L N, 'Research governance: current knowledge among clinical researchers', *Medical Journal of Australia*, 2008, 188: 649–52.

initiated by institutions, no data on the outcome of these investigations and no data on how often independent panels have been used. At present, it seems that the only way the general public or even the research community can learn about instances of alleged misconduct is when a dissatisfied whistle blower goes to the media.* Institutions in receipt of research funding from the NHMRC or the Australian Research Council (ARC) are obliged to notify the relevant funding agency when allegations of research misconduct have been received but this information is not made public.

The Australian Research Integrity Committee

A small reform step took place in 2011 when the NHMRC and the ARC jointly established the Australian Research Integrity Committee (ARIC).† I was appointed as one of the four inaugural members of ARIC. ARIC takes the form of a type of ombudsman. If a person is dissatisfied with how an institution has dealt with an allegation of research misconduct, that person can request that ARIC review the case. ARIC is not empowered to re-hear the matter; its role is to examine the process applied by the institution to determine whether the institution has abided by the guidelines set out in Part B of the *Australian Code for the Responsible Conduct of Research*. Reports of the findings and recommendations of ARIC in each case are sent to the CEO of either the NHMRC or the ARC to act on as each see fit. The

* Researchers might indirectly learn about alleged misconduct via a website dedicated to tracing retractions of scientific papers. See http://retractionwatch.com/.
† http://www.arc.gov.au/australian-research-integrity-committee-aric.

180

reports are confidential and thus I am not able to provide you any information about them. I can report that repeatedly ARIC reviews cases where institutions have allegedly failed to follow Part B of the Code and where conflicts of interest within the institution appear to have been ignored or badly handled. These failings generally tend to disadvantage the person who made the allegation of research misconduct (usually a junior researcher) and advantage the person against whom the allegation was made (usually a senior researcher/supervisor).

The *Australian Code* is presently being revised in a process that involves public consultation. The membership of the working party undertaking this task is drawn entirely from the university sector and there is no community representation. I fear that rather than strengthening Part B of the Code, it will be weakened in favour of the universities. In the meanwhile, concerned researchers and others have called for Australia to have the equivalent of the US Office of Research Integrity with the power to fully review the decisions taken by institutions dealing with allegations of serious research misconduct.[‡] Such a change will need significant political willpower to overcome the lobbying influences of universities. While I believe such an office is inevitable, I suspect that it will take public exposure of a major research misconduct scandal to generate the necessary political willpower for this to happen.

---

‡ Vaux D, 'From fraud to fair play: Australia must support research integrity', *Conversation,* 25 July 2013, https://theconversation.com/from-fraud-to-fair-play-australia-must-support-research-integrity-15733 and Breen, K J, 'Research misconduct – time for a rethink?', *Internal Medicine Journal*, 2016, 46: 728–33.

Lesser breaches should not be ignored

There are of course lesser breaches of the ethical framework surrounding research and the publication of research. One example remains imprinted on my mind. At our weekly hospital journal club, it was the turn of a senior clinician to present interesting recently published research papers. He explained that he had been too busy to prepare in the usual way and instead he chose to summarise for the group an unpublished manuscript that he had been asked to review by a journal editor. Needless to say, this was highly improper since in accepting to undertake the review he had expressly agreed that he would not show the manuscript to any other person without the permission of the editor. The attendees included several junior doctors and three or four other doctors engaged in research towards an MD or a PhD. My failure to speak up at the time effectively gave my approval to this ethical breach and may well have created the impression for the younger doctors that such conduct was acceptable. The only excuse that I can offer is that I dislike and shy away from personal confrontations. Perhaps I was so surprised by the behaviour as to be speechless but that is not a valid excuse. My only action was to leave the meeting as his presentation began, saying nothing.

While some might shrug their shoulders over minor breaches of the code of conduct for research and for the publication of research findings, in my view this is unwise. Accepting minor breaches, especially if they are repeated, carries the risk of creating an environment for researchers to be tempted to participate in more substantial breaches.

Chapter 12

DRUG COMPANIES AND THE MEDICAL PROFESSION

A yet to be resolved harmful relationship

Relationships between doctors and drug companies have long left me with a feeling of unease, but perhaps not as early in my career as they should have. As junior doctors, and even as medical students, we were invited to pharmaceutical trade displays at St Vincent's Hospital where every few months a number of drug companies mounted a one-day display of their products in a large room known as Brenan Hall. I went along and collected my share of various skin lotions, including corticosteroids, without the slightest hesitation. Much later, as director of the Gastroenterology Department, I resented the need to see representatives of these same companies but my resentment related to my not really having the time for them and my total failure to 'educate' the representatives who were very resistant to my interrupting their spiels with a different point of view. I felt obliged to see the representatives because I thought that, if I did not, our department might miss out on knowledge of new products and opportunities to participate in clinical trials.

During my time as director (1978–93), remarkable advances were made by a number of drug companies in creating new drugs which, for the first time, greatly reduced the amount of acid made by the human stomach and were generally free of side effects. At first, only gastroenterologists were authorised to prescribe these new drugs. As the sales of the drugs were spectacular, the companies did not lack funds to further promote their drugs to my colleagues, most often through gifts and offers to pay airfares to interstate and overseas medical conferences. By now, my concerns about this relationship were mounting. I felt that it was wrong but could not articulate why. However, I set my own rule by refusing any offer unless I was actually going to speak at a conference; i.e. I thought that since some work was involved in preparing, rehearsing and giving the talk, I was justified in receiving some recompense. Thus I can honestly report that only once in my career was my airfare paid by a drug company and that was to a conference in Brisbane celebrating the first five years of cimetidine (Tagamet) where I was a guest speaker in the 1980s. That came about because I was involved in a small trial of cimetidine compared to placebo in patients with erosive eosophagitis secondary to acid reflux. To the company's disappointment, the active drug proved no better than placebo.[*]

---

[*] Breen, K J, Desmond, P V and Whelan, G, 'Treatment of reflux oesophagitis. A randomised controlled evaluation of cimetidine', *Medical Journal of Australia*, 1983, 2: 555–6.

Another outcome of the industry being awash with money was the increased presence of drug companies at the annual conference of the Gastroenterological Society of Australia (a medical society formed in 1959 dedicated to the ongoing education of gastroenterologists). When I attended my first such conference in Brisbane in 1969, the conference was held at the University of Queensland, costs were kept to a minimum, there was no drug company sponsorship and every attending doctor paid his or her own way. In the 'PC' (post cimetidine) era, this all changed. Drug companies now became a central feature of the conferences. Conferences were no longer held in dingy university buildings but in upmarket hotels. Drug companies paid large fees to mount magnificent displays in a large hall set aside for trade displays. To ensure that every doctor could not avoid the displays (or avoid being pounced upon by company representatives), morning and afternoon coffee breaks and lunches were served in the trade display hall. It was not long before poster display sessions[†] were also held in the same room. Eventually, the annual conferences were so awash with money from drug companies that I stopped attending. The meetings now lasted a week and if one wanted to, one could get a 'free meal' and entertainment sponsored by a drug company every evening. I generally avoided such events and could usually find a few like-minded colleagues with whom to have dinner at our own expense (tax deductible of course!).

---

† Posters are a means whereby new clinical and laboratory research findings can be made available to registrants and the authors of the work are in attendance at set times to answer questions. They were introduced when the numbers of researchers wishing to give oral presentations outgrew the available time slots.

The gradual evolution of the influence of the industry

A very similar sequence occurred with a group of gastroenterologists in Melbourne. It is a story worth relating as it shows well the gradual evolution of the influence of the industry. I spent some time training in Sydney in 1969 and 1970 where I participated in regular evening educational meetings of a group of gastroenterologists known as the Sydney Gut Club. The meetings were held in hospitals and were free of industry sponsorship. After some time training in the USA, I returned to Melbourne in 1972 and with several colleagues arranged for an identical group to be called the Melbourne Gut Club. We met four times per year of an evening for a couple of hours of continuing education. For the first few years while I was the convenor/secretary, the meetings were held at major public hospitals on rotation. They were followed by a light supper which by agreement was restricted to 'hospital quality' sandwiches and tea or coffee and perhaps a glass of beer. The attendees were gastroenterologists and trainee gastroenterologists.

When a new convenor took over, it was decided that, for the last meeting of the year, there would be a dinner and that sponsorship from a drug company would be sought. This was readily forthcoming. The convenor had not thought through the planning as the first dinner was scheduled at a hotel in Queens Road in Albert Park with the Gut Club meeting to follow at nearby Prince Henry's Hospital. The dinner was a great success and much wine was drunk. As a result, only around half of the members came on to the meeting and some of those who did were not really in the mood for serious education. One of the presenters was a psychiatrist who spoke on possible links between constipation in infancy and the irritable bowel syndrome in adults. The less sober members of the audience entertained their neighbours with humorous and loud asides throughout the unfortunate man's talk. For the next few years, the Gut Club continued to hold a drug company sponsored annual dinner but it now followed the clinical meeting.

As this was the era of expanding drug company largesse, it was inevitable that a new convenor would accept offers from companies to provide a dinner after all four meetings each year. At that point, I stopped attending the dinners and only went to the clinical meeting component of the evening. Soon invitations to the dinners were extended to those nurses of each hospital who were now specialised as endoscopy nurses. The whole process had got out of hand in my view. I am pretty sure that most attendees felt that they were quite entitled to be given a free meal in an expensive restaurant four times a year.

Keeping their noses clean

Drug companies are much smarter than the collective medical profession. The companies seek to keep 'their noses clean' so that if or when their excesses in their relationships with doctors receive publicity there is the option of blaming the greedy doctors. Most gastroenterologists seek to attend the World Congress of Gastroenterology, a massive convention held in a handsome city every four years. I attended only two in my career, one in Mexico City in the 1970s and one in Sydney in 1990. At Mexico City, my impression was that drug company travel sponsorship was restricted to supporting a few delegates from developing nations, but by 1990 most gastroenterologists expected their travel costs would be met by a drug company. Even the companies began to be concerned about how this might look to the general public. In 1998, the World Congress was scheduled for Vienna, a very attractive venue. Most Victorian gastroenterologists I spoke with were keen to go and take their partners, especially if they could find a drug company that would pay for them. The company that was selling the biggest 'blockbuster' proton pump inhibitor (a very good drug for acid-related oesophageal reflux/heartburn) at the time was willing to do this and was offering a business class airfare (it may even have been two airfares but I now cannot recall). However, it seems that the company was concerned about adverse publicity should this generous support ever come to light. It instructed its representatives to inform each gastroenterologist they called on that this support was available but could only be released through the doctor writing to the company requesting travel assistance. The only possible reason for this new approach was to protect the company's reputation should adverse publicity arise; i.e. the blame could be attributed to greedy doctors. These were not under-paid GPs looking for help; these were mostly well-off gastroenterologists making a good income performing gastroscopies and colonoscopies in large numbers.

And here is another example of how smart the local pharmaceutical industry is. Until around the year 2000, the industry lobby group was known as the Australian

Pharmaceutical Manufacturers Association, an accurate name to my mind. Then, in a public relations coup, somebody had the idea to rebrand the lobby group as Medicines Australia! The equivalent lobby organisations in the UK and the USA meanwhile retain the non-misleading names of the Association of the British Pharmaceutical Industry and the Pharmaceutical Research and Manufacturers of America. I am sure that the average citizen hearing the name Medicines Australia would not imagine that this is the lobby organisation for Australia's drug manufacturers; more likely the name would conjure up some official government advisory body. Amazingly to me, the new name drew no adverse comments when it was first introduced. I still see it as a deliberately deceptive title. As described below, more recently the industry has again outwitted the regulators, sadly aided and abetted by the Federal AMA.

When I stepped down from being head of department in 1993, I ceased to see drug company representatives. The average proportion of doctors who see drug reps is around 80% but for specialists it is over 90%, so I was now in a very small minority. This decision gave me a great sense of relief and satisfaction but created an additional load on my secretary who had to keep the reps at bay. In making this decision, I mostly had my irritation with the spiels offered by drug reps as well as my own time and comfort in mind. I had never been unduly concerned that any contact could alter my prescribing habits. I was probably wrong about that, of course. Given the strength of the evidence (discussed below), it is highly likely that I too was subconsciously influenced by my contact with drug reps.

Finally taking a stance

It is worthwhile then to consider my 'Damascus' moment in this matter. At some point in 2003, it was my turn to present at our weekly journal club in the Department of Gastroenterology. In doing background reading for the new edition of our textbook, I had run across a paper written for an Australian psychiatric journal by Adelaide psychiatrist, Dr Jon Jurideini, and a colleague, Dr Peter Mansfield,* entitled 'Does drug promotion adversely influence doctors' abilities to make the best decisions for patients?'.† I was amazed to read all the evidence that was mounting that showed that the answer to this question was decidedly 'yes'. I felt that my gastroenterology colleagues needed to learn about this evidence so, rather than present a gastroenterological topic, I presented this paper to the journal club.

A little while later I read two equally powerful articles on the same topic published in the *British Medical Journal* written by Australian journalist and academic Ray Moynihan.‡ I was inspired to seek to try to bring all this disturbing material to the attention of Australian doctors more broadly and wrote a paper entitled 'The medical profession and the pharmaceutical industry – when will we open our eyes?' which was published in the *Medical*

* Dr Peter Mansfield is the founder and driving force behind the Australian based website Healthy Skepticism, http://www. healthyskepticism.org/global/.

† Published in *Australasian Psychiatry*, 2001, 9: 95–9.

‡ Moynihan, R, 'Who pays for the pizza? Redefining the relationships between doctors and drug companies. 1: Entanglement', *BMJ*, 2003, 326: 1189–92 and Moynihan, R, 'Who pays for the pizza? Redefining the relationships between doctors and drug companies. 2: Disentanglement', *BMJ*, 2003, 326: 1193–6.

Journal of Australia in mid-2004.§ My main message was that multiple studies from different countries and different health care systems have demonstrated how readily doctors' prescribing patterns can be influenced. These studies have shown that the more frequently a doctor sees a company representative, the more likely they are to prescribe inappropriately and the more likely they are to believe that they are not open to such influence. At that time, I was unaware of the important social science research published a year earlier which explained the subconscious influences at work.¶

My article in the *Medical Journal of Australia* gained some media attention but I was overseas when it appeared and was not interviewed. Two responses from leaders of the medical profession published in Australian print media revealed that getting doctors to appreciate that they were indeed susceptible to drug company promotions was going to be difficult. A vice-president of the Australian Medical Association was quoted as saying 'to simply presume prescribing habits are influenced by these companies is wrong' and the chair of the Australian Medical Association ethics committee was quoted as saying 'it was ridiculous to say that doctors were so easily influenced'. Thirteen years later, little had changed as in February 2017, the current AMA Federal president made similar remarks, while in August later that year, the AMA Federal vice president denied that 'there was any adverse impact on prescribing

§ Breen, K J, 'The medical profession and the pharmaceutical industry – when will we open our eyes?', *Medical Journal of Australia*, 2004, 180: 409–10.

¶ Dana, J, Lowenstein, G, 'A social science perspective on gifts to physicians from industry', *JAMA*, 2003, 290: 252–5.

behaviour arising from pharmaceutical company payments or educational events'.

Amazingly, between February 2017 and November 2017, the current AMA Federal President (to whom I had written on this subject on 17 February 2017) seems to also have had a 'Damascus moment'. In November he was quoted as telling the Newcastle Herald that 'Doctors should be aware of this influence and ensure their professional judgement is not compromised by industry relationships'. He informed AMA members that in the forthcoming revision of the AMA 2012 position statement on medical practitioners' relationships with industry, which 'did not specifically state that industry marketing can influence prescribing behaviour', this omission would be corrected.

The subconscious effects of industry promotions

There happen to be research-based explanations for why individual doctors accept the evidence that prescribing habits are influenced by drug companies yet fiercely believe that they are not so influenced. This seemingly illogical belief by most doctors puzzled me until I read this research. In summary, the answer to the puzzle is that the effects of gifts from drug companies are subconscious and so too is the closely related factor of self-interest. The effect of gifts, big or small, is based on the notion of developing relationships and generating (subconsciously) an obligation to reciprocate. It is difficult to refuse gifts, especially small gifts, as one does not wish to upset or offend the donor. Small gifts (pens, name plates and the like) are more than just simple reminders of the names of drugs or the companies. As doctors are not in the habit of giving gifts in return to drug representatives, the only way of reciprocating is to prescribe the company's product. Cleverly designed research shows that the impact of this exchange is subconscious, a finding which is completely consistent with the vigorous and at times angry denials that many doctors express when appraised of the well-documented effects on prescribing. Other psychological social research reveals that the influence of self-interest is also subconscious and powerful. As Dana and Lowenstein explained in their 2003 paper, this research shows that 'when individuals try to be objective, their judgements are subject to an unconscious and unintentional self-serving bias' and that 'small gifts may be surprisingly influential'.* Industry understands all this very well but as yet not many doctors seem willing to fully embrace the evidence.

Governments around the world responsible for funding health care are aware of the negative impact of drug company promotions (usually dressed up as 'education') and have sought to deal with the problem through a naming and shaming process. This began in the USA with some progressive states introducing legislation which was later adopted at the federal level in what became known as the 'Sunshine Act', i.e. shining light on the behaviour of doctors in the hope of changing it. Now in Australia, drug companies who are members of Medicines Australia are obliged to make public every six months the details of certain payments to doctors, covering such things as fees for speaking engagements, consultancies and advisory board

---

* Dana, J, Lowenstein, G, 'A social science perspective on gifts to physicians from industry', *JAMA,* 2003, 290: 252–5.

meetings, and sponsorship to attend educational events.[*] This reporting fails to capture the most common forms of interaction between doctors and industry, much to the delight of the Federal Australian Medical Association which proudly proclaimed on its website: 'The AMA supports transparency of pharmaceutical company relationships with practitioners. The AMA lobbied hard – starting in 2012 – to make sure a USA-style transparency system was not imposed in Australia. This would have required the collection of information about every industry-practitioner 'transaction' equal to or over $10 in value, such as providing tea and biscuits at a meeting'.[†]

The transparency claimed by Medicines Australia is a gross overstatement. The information that any patient might want to examine in regard to a particular doctor is extremely difficult to assemble. The lists of funds dispersed in the previous six months are provided separately for 37 individual drug companies so to track down payments to any individual doctor, a person would have to search 37 different data bases! I have no doubt that this design is deliberate. I am sure that Medicines Australia has no wish for the information to be more readily accessible. Indeed, the organisation probably assumes that members of the public will never look at the website.

There is an additional consequence with this approach that I predict. Because of the relatively narrow choice of the data placed on the website, it primarily relates to a selected group of specialist physicians and psychiatrists

* See Medicines Australia website https://medicinesaustralia.com. au/code-of-conduct/transparency-reporting/.
† https://ama.com.au/article/medicines-australia-new-code-con- duct-what-it-means-medical-practitioners.

who for good and not so good reasons work closely with the pharmaceutical industry. My anticipation is that many of this group will look at the data to see how they compare with their colleagues and will regard it as a badge of honour to be among the more highly remunerated. Even their patients, easily misled, might see this as evidence of their doctor's superior qualities.

If this prediction proves to be correct, it will have parallels with an earlier outcome of supposed transparency. At medical conferences around the world, it has become common practice for any medical specialist who is giving a lecture involving the use of drugs in the treatment of disease, or research into drugs, to show a slide listing all the drug companies from which that specialist has received support. This practice was introduced on the basis that through revealing such sponsorship, the audience members would somehow mentally adjust their interpretation of the data presented to allow for potential bias and conflicts of interest on the part of the speaker. There is no data to support this notion. Instead, many thoughtful people have suggested that the information has the opposite effect of adding to the credibility and aura of expertise of the speaker.

In case you are wondering, I have no problem with the argument that drug companies are an important component of our health care system and that through their investment in research, many significant advances in treatments have resulted. Sadly most doctors forget or overlook the fact that the prime responsibility of these companies is to their shareholders. As Katz and colleagues have written 'Drug companies are purely interested and invested in the products physicians prescribe, and they know and expect that their marketing will pay off with increased sales'. A former drug company CEO stated that marketing 'is almost as scientific as anything we do'. If the medical profession collectively ever admits there is a problem and agrees to try to do something about it, the focus should be on the education of doctors, seeking to alter their behaviour, and not on the conduct of the pharmaceutical industry.

The ethical issues involved

The ethical issues that surround how doctors deal with drug companies include the potential to undermine the trust that patients have in their doctors and the harm, mostly to the health care budget, that can be done by inappropriate prescribing. Patients universally assume that doctors will place the interests of their patients ahead of their own and trust that any advice or treatment provided will be independent of outside influences. For me it is depressing to observe how many doctors deny the influence of drug company advertising and promotions in the face of truly overwhelming evidence to the contrary. My medical colleagues cannot be excused forever for not taking this evidence on board.

Are there any mitigating circumstances? In defence of my colleagues, they are generally conscientious and caring doctors. Each genuinely believes that he or she is immune to the effect of advertising and promotion so they are not lying when they tell me this. They are clearly yet to appreciate that the industry's marketing effects are subconscious. On top of this, the gradual evolution of the clout of the drug industry has taken place over the last 40 to 50 years such that interactions with the industry are totally normalised. And as we have seen, there has been no leadership coming from the Australian Medical Association on this issue. The guidelines of the Australian Medical Association entitled *Medical Practitioners' Relationships with Industry 2010.* Revised 2012 actually support the use of industry funds; e.g. para 5.3.6 reads: 'Support for medical students, doctors-in-training and post-graduate fellows to attend educational events may be appropriate; however, the relevant organisation must be responsible for selecting the attendees as well as controlling the sponsorship funds'.* The guidelines issued by the Royal Australasian College of Physicians, guidelines now eleven years old, are equally permissive.†

The normalisation of strong interaction between drug companies and the medical profession begins during the medical student years. Drug companies know that this is of value to them even though students cannot prescribe drugs. And there is another group of health professionals now being targeted by industry – the new field of nurse practitioners who are able to prescribe certain drugs.

In my view more effort needs to be put into educating medical students and young doctors about the marketing techniques of industry and their influence (especially the subconscious influence) on prescribing habits. This must not just be by way of lectures but has to extend to role-modelling, stopping drug company access to these young people, and

---

* https://ama.com.au/position-statement/medical-practitioners-re-lationships-industry-2010-revised-2012.
† https://www.racp.edu.au/docs/default-source/advocacy-library/guidelines-for-ethical-relationships-between-physicians-and-in-dustry.pdf. These guidelines were under review as at March 2018.

banning company support for all educational events in our hospitals and medical schools.

Some pockets of resistance and change are emerging. In many US teaching hospitals, drug company representatives are banned and company access to medical students is precluded. At least one major medical association in the USA no longer seeks funding for its annual conferences from industry and here in Australia, the College of Emergency Medicine does not accept advertising from drug companies in its regular journal. While I was still in practice in the mid-2000s, the then CEO of St Vincent's Hospital, Melbourne responded very positively to my letter suggesting that the hospital fund a sandwich lunch that preceded the weekly medical grand rounds conference. Until then, lunch had been paid for by a different drug company each week, and as well, each company mounted a display of products and provided a representative to talk with those present. The attendees included junior doctors and medical students.

For the non-medical reader I will briefly summarise the ways in which drug companies usually interact with doctors or seek to promote their products with doctors. For the majority of doctors in clinical practice, contact occurs through face to face visits by drug company representatives, receipt of advertising material in the daily mail, reading medical journals and medical newspapers containing multiple advertisements, and attending drug company sponsored talks usually linked to a fine dinner. Studies have shown that the approach used by drug reps when visiting a doctor follows a very predictable pattern and includes giving gifts,[*] providing drug samples (also known as 'starter

---

[*] Gifts such as golf balls with logos on them and office items known

packs') and literature, issuing invitations to upcoming events, emphasising what medical opinion leaders have to say about any drug and describing how the doctors' peers are using the drug. To demonstrate the saturation of medical practices with drug reps, it has been estimated that in the USA there is one drug representative for every eight doctors and that an average of US$25,000 is spent per doctor per year on promotion, including medical education. The situation in Australia is likely to be very similar.[†] It is also estimated that the industry in the USA spends much more on marketing each year than it does on research and development.

The interactions between industry and selected specialists are more complex as specialists are often involved in conducting clinical trials of new drugs, presenting their findings to and sharing expertise with other groups of doctors in the role of what is now termed a 'key opinion leader', and serving as paid members of advisory boards for the drug companies.

And what about the pharmaceutical industry?

While focussing on the ethical and professional conduct of doctors (which is something that the medical profession should be able to address), I don't want to let the drug

---

as 'product reminders' are now banned. However, gifts in the form of educational items are still permitted. See https://medicine-saustralia.com.au/wp-content/uploads/sites/52/2010/01/20150617-PUB-Code-Edition-18-FINAL.pdf.

† Fabbri, A, Grundy, Q, Mintzes, B et al., 'A cross-sectional analysis of pharmaceutical industry-funded events or health professionals in Australia', *BMJ Open* 2017;7:e016701.doi:10.1136/bmjopen-2017-016701.

companies off the hook completely. The conduct of many of the large pharmaceutical companies has been the subject of several well researched books,* the most recent being that of Dr Peter Gøtzsche which is entitled *Deadly medicines and organised crime: How big pharma has corrupted healthcare.* Radcliffe Publishing, London, 2013. As I wrote in a review of Dr Gøtzsche's book for the *Medical Journal of Australia* in 2014:† 'This enlightening, alarming and depressing book deserves a wide readership among doctors but also among politicians, health administrators, and drug and medical device regulators. While there is no shortage of books that have sought to expose the misconduct of the pharmaceutical industry (one thinks of the books of Braithwaite, Kassirer, Angell, Moynihan and Goldacre), I finished this book with the feeling that things are getting worse and not better. The author is a Danish physician with expertise in clinical

---

* Other books worth reading on this topic include: Angell M, *The truth about drug companies: How they deceive us and what to do about it*. Random House, New York, 2004, pp. 37–51. Caplovitz A. *Turning medicine into snake oil. How pharmaceutical marketers put patients at risk*. NJPIRG Law and Policy Center, Trenton NJ, 2006. Goldacre B, *Bad pharma: How drug companies mislead doctors and harm patients*. Faber & Faber, London, 2013. Healy D. Pharmageddon. University of California Press, Oakland, 2013. Kassirer, J, *On the take: How medicine's complicity with big business can endanger your health*. Oxford University Press, New York, 2004. Moynihan, R, *Sex, lies and pharmaceuticals. How drug companies are bankrolling the next big condition for women*. Allen & Unwin, Sydney, 2010. Moynihan, R, Cassels, A, *Selling Sickness. How drug companies are turning us all into patients*. Allen & Unwin, Sydney, 2005. Welch, G, Schwartz, L, Woloshin, S, *Over-diagnosed: Making people sick in the pursuit of health*. Beacon Press, Boston, 2011.

† Breen K J. 'Deadly medicines and organised crime. How big pharma has corrupted healthcare', *Medical Journal of Australia*, 2014, 200 (6): 351. © Copyright 2014 *Medical Journal of Australia* – reproduced with permission.

trials and statistics, and earlier experience working in the pharmaceutical industry. He understands the need to substantiate the allegations he makes and uses extensive publicly available documentation covering at least 30 pharmaceutical companies. The book is well written and well planned with 22 chapters, each addressing discrete issues. This makes it easy to read and his arguments easy to follow.

His criticisms of the industry are wide-ranging. In early chapters, the author identifies fraudulent conduct by several big companies, many involving settlements of billions of dollars, and convincingly compares this conduct with the modus operandi of crime syndicates. Subsequent chapters address themes such as the impotence of drug regulators, lack of efficacy of many new drugs, concealment of clinical trial data including serious adverse effects, conflicts of interest at medical journals, alleged corruptive influence of drug company money, marketing disguised as clinical trials, creation of 'new' diseases, and his desire to bust industry myths. He also addresses industry exaggeration of the cost of developing new drugs, abuses of the rights of research participants, diminishing clinician input into trial design, conduct and reporting, and conflicted positions of clinicians who collaborate with industry and are paid in their roles as key opinion leaders.

The author seeks to identify root causes of these problems and blames in particular the dominance of the industry marketing arm in company management. He also highlights ineffectual regulation because governments now expect regulators to survive on industry funding. Finally, the book proffers several thoughtful suggestions for change, only two of which (improved access to data from all clinical trials and disclosure of industry payments to doctors) are likely to become widespread in the near future. Overall this book is a must read for all doctors in clinical practice.'

The behaviour of 'big pharma', especially in the USA, should be of concern to everyone. From my perspective, nothing will change so long as the companies facing legal action can arrange to pay huge settlements by way of fines rather than have executives sent to prison. For large companies that are making extraordinary profits, such settlements are probably regarded as the cost of doing business. As one example, in the USA GlaxoSmithKline pleaded guilty to criminal charges in 2012 and settled the matter by paying fines totalling $3 billion. This and many similar settlements by other companies are listed on an accessible website.[*]

For a more detailed description of the issues raised in this chapter, see Chapter 19 entitled 'Doctors, industry and conflicts of interest' in *Good Medical Practice: Professionalism, Ethics and Law*, 4th edn. published by the Australian Medical Council, Canberra 2016.

---

[*] http://en.wikipedia.org/wiki/List_of_largest_pharmaceutical_settlements_in_the_United_States.

Chapter 13

WHAT MAKES A GOOD DOCTOR

And how to identify one

What makes a good doctor is a subject now much discussed. It exercises those who are responsible for selecting young people to enter medical school and those responsible for turning new medical students into doctors. To date, the only thing that can be accurately predicted in selecting medical students is that high academic achievement identifies those most likely to graduate as doctors. Unfortunately, high academic achievers do not necessarily make good doctors.

In the fourth edition of our text book *Good Medical Practice: Professionalism, Ethics and Law*, we devoted a new chapter entirely to the topic of what constitutes a good doctor.[†] There we defined a good doctor as 'one who strives to practise competently, upholds the ethical standards of medicine, is committed to all the roles expected of doctors, is professional in his or her approach to clinical practice, is able to balance the 'art' and the 'science' of medicine and who at the same time maintains an appropriate balance

---

† Breen, K J, Cordner, S M and Thomson, C T, *Good Medical Practice: Professionalism, Ethics and Law*. Australian Medical Council, 2016, Kingston ACT. ISBN 978-1-938182-67-9.

between the professional and social spheres of daily life'. We acknowledged that being a good doctor twenty-four hours a day is very demanding. In the same chapter, we listed the various qualities that go to make a good doctor, a long list that included a capacity for self-reflection, compassion and empathy, fidelity, trustworthiness and integrity, veracity (truthfulness), respect for patients, discernment or judgement, collegiality and capacity for teamwork, willingness to serve patients and the community (altruism), and preparedness to be an advocate for the patient. Central to good medical practice are well-developed communication skills and there is a separate chapter in our textbook devoted to this. This long list of qualities and the preceding definition clearly represent an academic approach which is unlikely to hold the attention of, or be of assistance to, people seeking a new doctor as their general practitioner or people asking for the name of a good specialist.

So here I seek to address the question more pragmatically. What I hope to find in a really good doctor are the humanistic qualities of compassion, empathy and altruism. Of course, such doctors also need to be competent, up to date in their knowledge, thorough and conscientious. In straightforward consultations, it will usually not be necessary for these humanistic qualities to be overtly demonstrated, so are there markers that provide some hint of such underlying qualities? I suggest that patients should be able gain some insights into the character of any doctor from the doctor's attitude to communication, their being reasonably punctual, and their fees. Doctors who communicate well will introduce themselves by name, address you by name and look at you when inviting you into the consultation room. Good doctors will apologise if they are behind schedule, and inform you frankly about billing arrangements, especially if out of pocket expenses are involved. If out of pocket expenses are high, you can be confident of that doctor's lack of altruism. Gender can also make a difference as in the demonstration of the above qualities, and of good communication skills, I believe women doctors easily, but not universally, outperform their male counterparts.

Doctors who are good communicators listen to you without early interruption, make you feel comfortable in telling your story, help you to tell that story, avoid making you feel rushed, and provide feedback that gives you confidence that you have been heard and understood. When you leave the consultation, you are clear about what has been agreed and about any future steps, whether those steps be testing, starting treatment, specialist referral or some other plan. If things don't go according to what has been proposed, or your understanding of it, a good doctor will respond promptly, either in person or via a helpful staff member, to a phone call inquiry from you or your representative.

Sometimes, decisions about diagnosis or treatments offered can leave patients in a state of uncertainty. In these situations, patients may ask themselves about the value of obtaining a second opinion but will hesitate to voice that question for fear of upsetting the doctor. In my view this is another means of assessing whether you are in the hands of a good doctor. A good doctor will welcome such a question and will facilitate you getting such an opinion. A really good doctor will anticipate the question and suggest a second opinion. Should a doctor be angered or appear irritated by such a request, you are not in the presence of a good doctor and you should go back to your GP and ask to be referred elsewhere.

Potential patients are easily misled by information about doctors they can find on the internet. The more glowing the description of qualifications, skills, hospital appointments and testimonials, the more sceptical one should be. Be very wary of those whose fees are well beyond average as there is no correlation of high fees with skill and ability; indeed, there may be an inverse correlation. High fees are simply evidence of what the market will bear.

It can be deeply frustrating if your GP refers you to a specialist and you find that there is a long wait to get an appointment. Should this happen you should go back and talk to your GP. If your GP feels that your problem is urgent, the GP can usually arrange for you to be seen earlier by contacting the specialist's office on your behalf. If the specialist is truly very busy and can't fit you in, the better ones will suggest the name of a trusted colleague. If your GP shrugs his or her shoulders and indicates that the situation cannot be helped, change your GP as soon as possible.

Good GPs should have some idea about the fees charged by the specialists they are referring you to. Patients should not hesitate to ask about this. A good GP will be happy to try to answer your questions. A bad GP will tell you to ask the specialist. When I was in practice as a specialist, it was not unusual for me as a medical specialist to refer patients to surgical specialists. I routinely sought feedback from patients about their experience, including out of pocket expenses. If the feedback was negative, that surgical specialist was removed from my list. I believe that good GPs should have the same approach but I have no insight into how common this is.

Another means of judging a good GP (and a good specialist) is via their attitude to providing repeat prescriptions for people with chronic (meaning longstanding) stable conditions.* Doctors who regularly insist that you attend for a consultation to receive a repeat prescription, or who bill you for a prescription that you collect from the receptionist without seeing the doctor, are greedy and not altruistic. Be aware, however, that there can be valid reasons which are in your best interests for the doctor to insist on seeing you. Where such reasons exist, a good doctor will take the trouble to explain them. A similar judgement about lack of altruism may be applied to doctors who charge for forwarding copies of your medical records when you change to another medical practice.

The professional standards expected of doctors

The professional standards expected of doctors are now spelt out in a national guideline known as 'Good medical practice: a code of conduct for doctors in Australia'.† Although prepared primarily by the medical profession through the state and territory medical boards and the Australian Medical Council, the working party had significant health consumer input and there was wide public consultation in its development. A key concern of health consumers on the

* A frequent error of journalists is to misuse or misunderstand the use of the adjectives 'acute' and 'chronic' in medicine. Acute appendicitis refers to the sudden onset of the illness and not to its severity. Similarly, a chronic illness refers to one that is persistent or likely to be longstanding. A chronic illness may be mild or severely disabling or anything in between.
† It is available to the public at http://www.medicalboard.gov.au/Codes-Guidelines-Policies/Code-of-conduct.aspx.

working party was their desire that doctors be consistently respectful of patients. The code of conduct is written in accessible language and deserves to be better known by the public. In the abstract, it is unlikely that many doctors would wish to argue with the standards set by the code. Sadly, less competent doctors often lack self-insight and hence are more likely to deny that their professional conduct is inconsistent with the code.

I place the capacity to empathise with patients as the most important quality of a good doctor. This quality can at times be a handicap as misplaced empathy can lead to inappropriate prescriptions or unreliable medical certificates. Competent doctors who exhibit empathy and altruism are over represented in the number of doctors who suffer from problems such as burn out, stress-related anxiety and depression, substance misuse with addiction, and relationship breakdown. This emphasises how difficult it can be to be a good doctor and is a further argument for well-funded doctors' health services as we need to strive to keep these doctors well, happy, and at work (see Chapter 6).

Over many years of observing trainee doctors and my peers in the workplace (i.e. in my case, in hospitals), I developed my own rule of thumb to identify doctors who were likely to be compassionate, altruistic and humble. It is a guide that mostly can't be used by patients which is a pity. I took notice of how each doctor related to the other hospital staff they encountered, be they nurses, secretaries, domestic staff or their own peers. Most doctors treated their peer doctors with courtesy and respect so this was not a useful differentiation. Most, but by no means all, senior doctors treated junior doctors with respect, at least while senior colleagues were present. However, many doctors, senior and junior, ignored the nurses, secretaries, domestic staff and others they worked with on a daily basis, not bothering to acknowledge their presence let alone find out and use their names. I mentally marked these doctors down and assumed that this apparent lack of respect translated to arrogance, aloofness and a poor attitude to communication when working with patients.

For those involved in the education and training of young doctors, questions arise as to whether empathy can be taught and whether young minds can be moulded to meet the requirements to be a good doctor. Overall, I am optimistic about the answers to these questions but suggest that the effects required must come mostly from role-modelling and mentoring and not just from the class room or text books. My optimism is tempered by two countervailing trends. First, in our teaching hospitals, and perhaps in general practices that take trainee doctors, time and cost pressures have reduced the opportunities for young doctors to observe at first-hand how experienced doctors talk with and care for patients and their families. Second, while there is good evidence that professionalism can be taught, I worry that this might be less effective in those who now enter medical school at a later age. This has come about with the move to graduate entry medical schools which require applicants to complete an initial university degree. I identify strongly with the remarks of the late American medical educator and ethicist, Dr Edmund Pellegrino, who wrote in 2002: 'Character formation cannot be evaded by medical educators. Students enter medical school with their characters partly formed. Yet, they are still malleable as they assume roles and models on their way to formation as physicians.'*

Is medicine a science or an art?

Another important question that has arisen in medical education in recent years is the question as to whether medicine is a science or an art. We reviewed the available opinion on this in Chapter 2 of our 2016 textbook.† This question has arisen because of the remarkable advances in medicine over the last seventy years, advances based in scientific methods, leading some to wish to depict medicine as a pure science. These amazing advances have brought new problems including rising health care costs, accusations of inappropriately extending life in older patients with terminal illnesses, and a sense that the whole person is not always considered when treatments are offered. The last problem may be exacerbated by technological advances that have contributed to fragmenting the medical profession into narrower and narrower specialties.

In my mind medicine is both an art and a science, best defined as the art of interpreting all the relevant circumstances of a patient, so as to decide, with the patient, how best to apply medical science.‡ If medicine is partly an art then how best can the art be taught and learnt? Some of the requirements such as communication skills can be

---

* Pellegrino, E D, 'Professionalism, profession and the virtues of the good physician', *Mount Sinai Journal of Medicine*, 2002, 69: 378–84.

† Breen, Cordner and Thomson, *Good Medical Practice*.

‡ Kaldjian, L C, 'Teaching practical wisdom in medicine through clinical judgement, goals of care, and ethical reasoning', *J Med Ethics*, 2010, 36: 558–62.

taught and practised but I believe that the essential means of teaching the art of medicine is to provide mentoring and good role-modelling of humanism by practising doctors in the traditional apprenticeship model. Anyone who believes otherwise has no understanding of what good medical practice entails.

The change to later (graduate) entry to medical school commenced in Australia when Sydney University went down this path in the 1990s. The change not only involved later entry but the course was also shortened from six to four years. This change was driven by a desire to avoid enrolling immature young people who sometimes realised part way through a six-year course that they were not suited to a career in medicine. Dropping out at that stage carried a high price as the student would not have a degree despite completing three or four years at university. An additional factor was to seek to ensure that the spectrum of people enrolled to study medicine roughly matched the make-up of the community the new doctors were to serve. I have not taught in a four-year course but there must be significant pressure on students and teachers to cover all the essential material. I am not aware of any comparisons of new graduates from the graduate entry courses and traditional six year courses. If there are any material differences, hopefully they will disappear after the additional five and more years of supervised training that general practitioners and specialists are required to undertake in Australia.

My alma mater, the University of Melbourne, also recently transitioned to a graduate entry program. It is based on the new 'Melbourne model' where all professional courses including medicine, law, engineering, dentistry, commerce etc. are graduate entry; i.e. anyone school leaver enrolling at the University of Melbourne is required to first complete a three-year undergraduate degree before progressing to their desired professional course. The medical faculty advises potential medical students to choose the undergraduate degree entitled Bachelor of Biomedicine during which students undertake detailed study of requisite subjects including anatomy, physiology and biochemistry. I find this development amusing as the full course (including the three-year undergraduate degree and the four-year MD graduate degree) strongly resembles the six-year course that I completed over fifty years ago – but it now takes seven years. So much for progress!

I am also critical of the new MD course at the University of Melbourne for what I see as an undue emphasis on research training and experience. All medical students are obliged to spend 'a semester in which each student is immersed in a single medical discipline to complete a research project'. I acknowledge that medical students need to acquire knowledge and insight into how laboratory and clinical research is central to improvements in health care but I believe that this time compulsorily spent in 'hands on' research is inappropriate and irrelevant to the needs of most medical graduates. Melbourne University's leaders seem to have overlooked that the primary reason for the university being granted the privilege of educating doctors (including the privilege of access for their students to patients in our public hospitals) is to provide the next generation of good doctors for the people of Victoria and Australia. I understand that some medical graduates will be attracted to a career in medical research and that these people are vitally important. However, to try to motivate every medical graduate to follow this path seems wasteful and indeed may be driven by the attraction of the extra pairs of hands the students provide in the university's research laboratories, at no cost. Hopefully a review of this aspect of the course, informed by student feedback, may lead to modification of this experiment. School leavers are 'voting' with their feet as Monash University's more traditional undergraduate medical degree has become more popular than the course at the University of Medicine, as assessed by the required ATAR (Australian Tertiary Admission Rank) score.

Chapter 14

THE NATIONAL SCHEME FOR REGULATING DOCTORS

An unsatisfactory situation

The national scheme for the registration and regulation of all health professionals, introduced in 2010, has only one redeeming feature to my mind and that is the portability of registration between the states and territories. And the single register now prevents disgraced doctors moving to practise interstate. Portability of registration is a significant benefit for those doctors who transfer interstate and for the 10% of doctors who regularly practise in more than one jurisdiction or across state borders. However, the national scheme has failed to win the confidence of the community and the medical profession and in some aspects has taken the regulatory process backwards. Many of the problems with the scheme were predictable.* In this chapter, I describe my view of the key elements of an effective system of regulation

* Breen, K J, 'National registration legislative proposals need more work and more time', *Medical Journal of Australia,* 2009, 191: 464–5 and Breen, K J, 'Doctors' health: Can we do better under national registration?', *Medical Journal of Australia,* 2011, 194: 191–2.

and then explore what is wrong with the national scheme and what might be required to improve it.

An effective regulatory scheme

First, what does an effective regulatory scheme look like? I frankly admit that when I took over as President of the Medical Practitioners Board of Victoria in 1994, I had not thought through many of these issues and it is only now in hindsight that I believe that I can see what works well and what is important. Indeed, without the new national scheme to contrast this with, I may never have crystallised my thinking. I now see that an effective regulatory scheme needs to have, or to develop, a number of key characteristics. These include a strong sense of trust, accessibility and responsiveness as seen by those who are regulated (i.e. the doctors) and those who are to be protected from harm (i.e. the community). Although the central reason for having a medical board is to protect the community from incompetent, poorly performing or impaired doctors, this protection is enhanced where the board is also trusted by the medical profession. For this reason, I will first discuss what I think are some key steps in gaining the trust of the profession.

In no particular order, the steps include adequate communication with the profession at large and with its various representative organisations, visibility and accessibility to the profession, and demonstration of respect for any doctor who is subject to being notified to the Board. The new Medical Practitioners Board of Victoria from 1994 put time and resources into communicating with the profession, especially via a printed bulletin issued regularly, but also by sending every doctor a printed copy of the Board's annual report. While the bulletin may not have been read by all recipients, anecdotal evidence told us that there was considerable interest in its content, which included summaries of all formal hearings as well as summaries of some informal hearings selected for their educational value. As informal hearings were not open to the public, the names and any identifying aspects of the doctors involved were not provided.

The Board also made efforts to communicate regularly with key medical organisations including AMA Victoria and the Victorian medical indemnity organisations. Board staff were provided with communication training to ensure that doctors approaching the Board or contacted by the Board were dealt with respectfully. Staff were reminded that for the individual doctor, contact with the Medical Board could be a very stressful experience. As president, I made myself available to speak with any doctor who sought to contact me, as did other members of the Board.

Another means of communicating with the medical profession was the manner in which each year the new cohort of medical graduates from Victoria's medical schools were registered and welcomed into the profession. While each graduate was required to attend the Board's office to complete all the necessary paper work, the actual registration was a formal event held a day or so after their university graduation ceremony. For this the Board members travelled to the medical school campus. Here new registrants assembled in a large lecture theatre and the individual Board members were introduced by name and professional background. Then following some words of welcome from the President, two or three Board members spoke briefly to the new doctors about the various responsibilities that came with registration, about the importance of maintaining a healthy work-life balance and about common problems that should and could be avoided. Following this group session, each registrant met individually with a Board member who signed and presented their certificate of registration.

To seek to foster trust and confidence in the Board's processes, the Board employed two experienced doctors as its part-time investigating officers. Their role was to investigate and make an initial assessment of complaints made against doctors and then present their findings and recommendations in person to the Board. I felt that the use of experienced doctors was critical for the evaluation of any complaint as it meant that the doctor being investigated could have confidence that the account of events and the surrounding clinical circumstances would be more readily appreciated. While we did not set time limits or targets for the completion of any investigation, the fact that the investigating officers were employed directly by the Board, attended the fortnightly meetings of the Board and were generally accessible whenever I was at the Board, meant that delays were very unusual. I was deeply disappointed when I learned that, after I retired from the Board, these doctors were replaced by other health professionals, apparently as a cost-saving measure.

The establishment of the Victorian Doctors Health Program (see Chapter 6) was another means of increasing the trust of the medical profession in the Board as the Program demonstrated the Board's genuine concern to see that doctors who were unwell and at risk of becoming impaired were provided with early and non-threatening access to high quality care and later, if needed, assistance to return to work.

Gaining the trust of the community is a much larger issue. In my view, it hinges on treating every complainant with the utmost respect, dealing with complaints as promptly and fairly as possible, and maintaining open communication when matters take longer than usual to resolve. For the most vulnerable complainants, we took additional trouble. Hence, as discussed in Chapter 7, the Board employed a highly qualified female investigating officer to handle sexual misconduct complaints and we established an independent service to support complainants through the stresses of giving evidence at formal hearings.

As community trust is also built by what is published in the media, the new Board was proactive in this regard. Formal hearings were announced in the law lists that appeared in the daily papers and I made myself available to talk to the media when asked. Another element of trust is the relationship with the Minister of Health to whom the Board was responsible. This meant not only being available to answers questions and attend meetings as requested but also being proactive to alert the Minister's office should a contentious issue be on the horizon.

What are the problems with the new national scheme?

With that background, I will now turn to the new national scheme of medical regulation. Most doctors are unaware that the system introduced in 2010 is not truly a national scheme. From the outset, New South Wales chose to almost fully opt out to become what is euphemistically called a co-regulated jurisdiction. It kept its own Medical Board, renaming it the Medical Council of NSW. Three years later, Queensland also chose to be co-regulated.

For the other states and territories that are in the scheme, the regulation of doctors is divided between the Australian Health Practitioner Regulation Agency (AHPRA) and the Medical Board of Australia (MBA). The MBA is the over-arching national body which sets policy and issues guidelines for the medical profession. Then there are state and territory medical boards (i.e. local branches of the MBA) that handle professional conduct and health issues and the like. Complaints about doctors and notifications under the mandatory reporting laws are investigated by non-medical staff employed by, and responsible to, AHPRA. The results of those investigations are passed to the state medical board where decisions are made as to the disposition of each complaint. When that disposition is to refer allegations of serious misconduct to a formal hearing, the hearing is conducted by a separate state-based tribunal. For example, in Victoria this is the Victorian Civil and Administrative Tribunal.

There is a long list of what is wrong with the national scheme for the regulation of the medical profession. What follows is a summary; I have written in more depth elsewhere.* The scheme embraces fourteen health professions

* See: Breen, K J, 'National registration scheme at five years: not what it promised', *Australian Health Review*, 2016, 40(6): 674–8 and Breen, K J, 'What ails the national registration scheme for Australia's 600,000 health professionals?', http://johnmenadue.com/

but for simplicity and because of my perspective, I have only addressed the issues as I see them for doctors. Some of the problems reside in the legislation while others can be attributed to the structure and implementation of the scheme. Many of these problems have been hidden from the public and have not often been the subject of media attention. Given that in its first six years of operation, the scheme has been the subject of three Federal parliamentary inquiries and one state parliamentary inquiry, this is surprising to say the least.

As already pointed out, this is not truly a national scheme. The largest jurisdiction, New South Wales, which has 32% of Australia's doctors, never joined the scheme. The renamed NSW Medical Council continues all its pre-2010 roles with the exception of managing the registration of doctors. Registration is handled by a small NSW branch office of the Medical Board of Australia. The absence of NSW doctors from the system has had implications for all of Australia's doctors because the largest subgroup of doctors in the country is basically unaware of the problems with a scheme that does not involve them. I suggest that this lack of involvement and concern has had an impact on the interest of the Federal AMA in the scheme and its capacity to make its views heard by health ministers.

To compound the situation, within three years of the commencement of the national scheme, the third largest jurisdiction, Queensland, with 20% of Australia's doctors, also chose to become a 'co-regulated' state. So now more than half of Australia's doctors are not part of the so-

blog/?p=6150. These papers contain links and references to a large number of relevant sources of information.

called national scheme. An inquiry commenced in 2012 by a committee of the Victorian Parliament recommended that Victoria, with 25% of Australia's doctors, should also opt for co-regulation. Unfortunately, in my view, this recommendation was not acted upon.

The new system was undoubtedly rushed in its implementation. Nobody has ever explained why this was so. My guess is that the bureaucrats and politicians leading the process were fearful that if the process was delayed, it might fall over completely. The legislation that drives the scheme is called the 'national law' but this is not legislation of the Federal Parliament. Instead it is a series of state and territory laws that, through an agreement reached via the COAG Health Council (a gentlemen's agreement, as it is not binding), are based on a law first passed by the Queensland Parliament. The choice of Queensland was undoubtedly because its Parliament is unicameral so there was no upper house that might insist on modifications to the legislation, as later occurred in Western Australia.

Through being rushed, there were teething problems in the first year of transition, when the existing state registration data bases needed to be merged. Large numbers of doctors and other health professionals found themselves unregistered through no fault of their own. Confidence in the new system was undermined from the start and probably has never recovered. In the lead up to the new scheme, doctors were promised that there would be efficiencies of scale and that this would help to keep the costs of registration down. This promise was not kept as in 2010, the fee for annual renewal of medical registration in Victoria rose from $410 to over $600. Similar increases were seen in every jurisdiction.

This was a very bad outcome as the interim agency that was responsible for developing the national scheme had assured doctors of cost savings. This was yet another blow to the confidence that the medical profession needed to have in the system.

As mentioned, there are problems with the legislation as well as problems in the structure and reporting relationships of the scheme. Of course the structure and reporting relationships are driven partly by the legislation, but with regard to the distinct aspects of the legislation that impact on the confidence that doctors need to have with the scheme, there are at least three problems.

Most troubling is Section 141 of the national law which covers mandatory reporting of several forms of alleged misconduct such as sexual misconduct and also covers mandatory reporting of allegedly impaired ill doctors 'where that impairment has placed the public at risk of substantial harm'. In my view, it is unnecessarily stigmatising to include the reporting of ill-health with the reporting of allegations of sexual misconduct; ill-health and associated possible impairment should be dealt with separately in the national law. If this had been done from the start, the much more troubling problem with mandatory reporting could have been identified and avoided. That problem is that the mandatory reporting obligation applies to treating doctors. It creates a deterrent to doctors seeking help. Even the Medical Board saw the problem and tried to help by issuing advice about the application of the law. This advice may have only compounded the difficulty treating doctors were having in interpreting the law. If the Medical Board really understood the issues involved and was serious about gaining the confidence of the medical profession, the Board should have publicly declared that the section of the legislation was potentially harmful and directly lobbied the health ministers for an amendment.

What I found very frustrating about this section of the law is that it should never have become a problem in the first place. As I wrote in 2009 before the national law was finalised 'The draft legislation will set back improvements in recent years with earlier presentation of sick doctors and improved access to best available help. It goes far beyond the modern legislation in most Australian jurisdictions in at least three ways; it extends the statutory reporting obligation to all doctors and not just treating doctors; it fails to separate illness from possible impairment; and it fails to identify that any possibly impaired doctor who agrees voluntarily to suspend practice is no longer a risk to the public and should not be reported to a medical board. If an existing template has been used, the obvious source is the 2008 mandatory reporting amendments to the NSW *Medical Practice Act*. However, those amendments do not extend to doctors who may be practising while impaired; in NSW such reporting remains an ethical and professional obligation'.* Mine was never a lone voice in the debate about mandatory reporting of alleged impairment due to illness. Similar concerns were expressed at a Senate inquiry in 2009 before the 'national law' was finalised[†] and at a further Senate inquiry in 2011.[‡]

* Breen, K J, 'National registration legislative proposals need more work and more time', *Medical Journal of Australia,* 2009, 191: 464–5.
† https://www.aph.gov.au/Parliamentary_Business/Committees/Senate/Community_Affairs/Completed_inquiries/2008-10/registration_accreditation_scheme/report/index.
‡ https://www.aph.gov.au/Parliamentary_Business/Committees/Senate/Finance_and_Public_Administration/Completed_inqui-

It took seven years for the health ministers to finally agree that this was a problem. Sadly, the recognition of the problem was driven by a spate of suicides by young doctors. All that was needed to overcome the problem was to extend to other jurisdictions a Western Australian amendment to the national law that relieved treating doctors of the legal duty to report impaired doctors who posed a risk to the public but did not excuse them from their ethical duty in this regard. Instead the health ministers chose to seek a more complex solution meaning that mandatory reporting was still in place as at April 2018.

Another troubling element of the national law is Section 178. This section empowers the Medical Board to caution a doctor over alleged poor professional performance without that doctor being interviewed by an investigating officer or a Board member. Under Section 206, there is an obligation for any employer to be informed of such a caution, with the attendant implication that something unprofessional has taken place. Yet, under Section 199, such a caution cannot be appealed whereas all other Board decisions can be appealed. These sections must be amended.

A third problem with the national law was that it failed to define what was meant by the term '*clinical practice*'. Because of this, doctors who had recently retired from clinical practice, and who had chosen non-practising registration, were left very uncertain as to whether such registration allowed them to perform roles such as teaching and mentoring. In response to this uncertainty the Medical Board issued its own definition of clinical practice. This definition proved to only increase the uncertainty and in response to further criticism,

ries/2010-13/healthpractitionerregistration/index.

the Board then issued an interpretation of its definition. This multitude of problems meant that from early in its existence the Board struggled to gain the confidence of the medical profession.

In regard to the structural problems, the key issues include ministerial oversight; divided responsibilities; complexity involved in amending the national law; the independence of investigative staff (employed by AHPRA) from the Medical Board, with a consequent lack of accountability; the size and remoteness of the massive bureaucracy that has been created; and the relative invisibility of the state and territory medical boards that actually do the work of interacting with the medical profession. Yet, it has not been these problems that have been the main focus of parliamentary inquiries. These inquiries to a certain extent have sought to address community concerns over the efficiency of complaint handling and poor communication. Thus not only has the national scheme failed to win the confidence of doctors but it has also failed to win community confidence. I don't blame the staff of AHPRA or the various members of the medical boards, as I think that they have mostly tried their best. They are simply saddled with a badly thought out system that is not suitable for Australia.

Let me look at these structural issues in more depth, starting with the chain of responsibility of health ministers. Under the previous state-based medical board structure, each board was directly responsible to the local parliament via the state or territory health minister. Under the national scheme, if a health minister has a concern, that concern has to be first raised with all the other health ministers around the country and agreement sought on what action if any is to be taken. If agreement is reached, the ministers then need to communicate not only with the relevant national board but also with AHPRA and AHPRA's committee of management. This is a recipe for lack of responsibility and of responsiveness as no one health minister is in charge of the system.

Should the ministers agree that the national law needs to be amended, new obstacles arise as eight different parliaments need to pass the proposed amendments as agreed. As some parliaments have an upper house, there is no guarantee that agreed amendments will pass through eight parliaments unscathed. The valuable Western Australian amendment to the mandatory reporting provisions attests to the power of an upper house. In the long term, maintaining a single national law will be problematic. More importantly the system we now have may prove to be inflexible and unable to be altered in response to changing circumstances.

Divided responsibilities are already implied by the above discussion of ministerial responsibility but this extends much further. It is not clear in any issue that arises for the medical profession whether the Medical Board of Australia is in charge of its own affairs or whether the final arbiter is AHPRA. As the national scheme is designed to provide uniform regulatory conditions for all fourteen health professions which are included, the Medical Board can rarely 'go it alone'. Instead as policy is developed, the other thirteen boards have to be consulted. Even if the outcomes are satisfactory, this at the very least is a recipe for delay and also for reaching the lowest common denominator.

I have earlier mentioned how under the previous state-based system, investigative staff were appointed by and accountable to the medical board. Divided responsibilities under the national scheme have altered this accountability as investigative staff are employed by and are accountable to AHPRA. This has had many practical downsides. Well over half the investigative staff are not health professionals and none to my knowledge are medical practitioners. This change is guaranteed to diminish the confidence that doctors need to have in the regulator. I am very aware of the consequences of this change as I have repeatedly counselled doctors who have been distressed by the insensitive handling of complaints by AHPRA staff. From these experiences, I have gained a sense that the starting point for some investigative staff is to assume that the doctor is in the wrong (guilty until proven innocent). While dissatisfied doctors can take their issues up with the federal health ombudsman's office, this is rarely used, partly because one is obliged to first lodge a complaint with AHPRA, and partly through fear of repercussions should the doctor ever have to deal with AHPRA again. Once again, here is a system that doctors cannot have confidence in.

The national registration scheme is a massive undertaking. In its annual report, AHPRA's main emphasis is on numbers as it registers over 600,000 health professionals. This size is one of its downfalls as is shown by its annual report. This voluminous electronic document covering fourteen health professionals is almost certainly not read by most doctors. The educational value that may have attached to previous annual reports directed at a single profession and jurisdiction has been completely lost. Another aspect of the AHPRA annual report, and of the electronic bulletins that emerge from the Medical Board of Australia, is the relative invisibility of each state and territory medical board. Without any sense of familiarity with local board members it is more difficult to maintain a sense of confidence in the board.

Finally, there are two other aspects of the national scheme that I suggest are clearly a waste of resources. I refer first to the requirement that every year, each national board is obliged to negotiate a 'health profession agreement' with AHPRA. Section 25 of the national law states that a central function of AHPRA is 'to provide administrative assistance and support to the National Boards and the Boards' committees in exercising their functions'. In practice, it appears to me that AHPRA, via its administrative staff, dictates to the Medical Board and its state Medical Board branches (committees) what work is done on behalf of the Boards as well as its quality and timeliness. To gain access to this 'administrative assistance and support', the Medical Board of Australia has to spend time and resources every year negotiating a budget for its supply. What a waste!

I am critical of the process by which the national medical accreditation body, the Australian Medical Council, is engaged by the Medical Board. The effect of a one-size fits all health professions approach taken with the national law has led to recurrent uncertainty and a waste of resources for the Australian Medical Council. In the report of the Productivity Commission that led to the national scheme, it was recommended that any accreditation agency should be separate from the registration agency. However, under the national law, the accreditation arm is part of, and subservient to, the national registration board. This has the effect for the Australian Medical Council of having to, from time to time, make a detailed application to the Medical Board of Australia to request that it be reappointed as the accreditor of medical schools and medical colleges. Not only is this a waste of time and energy but it is demeaning to an accreditation agency that is respected internationally and has become an icon in Australian medicine. This is another section of the national law that should be amended.

What should be done?

So, what should be done overall? Given the complexity and size of the national scheme, as well as the very strong case for having portable national registration and agreed national legislation, I do not suggest that the system should be completely dismantled. The experimental national scheme can rightfully claim that it has successfully established a single national register and, with it, ready portability of registration across Australia. I therefore suggest that national registration and maintenance of the national register must continue and that this task should remain with AHPRA. For all other medical board functions, including complaint handling and investigation, professional performance assessment and disciplinary hearings, and assessment of health/impairment issues, I recommend that every jurisdiction should opt to copy NSW and become co-regulatory. If co-regulation can work effectively for NSW which has 32% of Australia's 103,000 doctors and 27% of Australia's 370,000 nurses, it should be abundantly clear that a single national register can work similarly with all the other state and territory medical boards becoming co-regulated entities.

Chapter 15

STILL TILTING AT WINDMILLS

And not always winning

While I retired from all clinical practice at the end of 2008, I did not cease to think about the well-being of my medical colleagues and the medical profession generally nor about the issues that arise in medical regulation, medical ethics, medical indemnity insurance and related areas. I served as chairman of the Board of the Victorian Doctors Health Program from 2005 to 2009, as a part-time member of the Federal Administrative Appeals Tribunal from 2006 to 2014 and as Commissioner of Complaints for the NHMRC from 2007 to 2013. In 2011, I was appointed as one of the inaugural members of the Australian Research Integrity Committee. From the time of retiring from clinical practice in 2008 through until 2016, I also regularly spent time keeping up to date with all aspects of the contents of our textbook. Partly as a result of these interests and partly through my past experiences, I found it impossible to resist joining in many of the debates and discussions of issues confronting the medical profession.

Many of these issues have already been canvassed in earlier chapters. Here I cover a few more, in an order that neither reflects my sense of their importance to the profession nor the temporal relationships of the issues.

The Federal Administrative Appeals Tribunal

From my seven years as a part-time member of the Federal Administrative Appeals Tribunal (AAT), I became much more aware of the important role that the AAT plays (in my non-legal language) in acting as a safety barrier against ill-judged or wrong decisions made by the administrative arm of government (i.e. government department staff and at times the relevant minister). As a medically qualified member without a legal degree, I only heard appeals that had a significant medical content, primarily appeals against decisions of Centrelink, the Department of Veterans Affairs and Comcare (the Commonwealth workers compensation scheme), sometimes sitting on my own, but more often with a legally qualified member.

One thing that frequently struck me was the inability of expert medical witnesses (with a few notable exceptions) to present their reports or give oral evidence without prejudice, even when questioned by the Tribunal (i.e. yours truly). For many such witnesses, it was readily apparent that they avoided answers that might conflict with the arguments being mounted by the law firm or government department that had paid for their reports. This effect may well be subconscious, akin to the effect of drug company promotions. If an expert medical witness is confident and presents well and if the witness is not cross-examined thoroughly, there is a risk that a legally qualified tribunal member, not sensitive to this bias, might be unduly swayed by what is heard. For this reason alone I hope that, despite budget stringencies, the AAT continues to have medically qualified members appointed to it.

AAT members do not have the protection of permanent appointments and reappointment is at risk of political influence. Members are appointed by the Federal Attorney-General. Both major political parties can be accurately accused of making partisan appointments. The President of the AAT for half of my time as a member was Attorney-General in a previous ALP federal government. In 2017, the then Attorney-General, Mr George Brandis, was accused of making political appointments and of not reappointing members who had been involved in making decisions with which Federal ministers were unhappy. In the subsequent uproar, politicians got away with criticisms of the AAT that were wrong and misleading. Serving members were unable to respond publicly but former members were not so constrained. Former member, Mr John Handley, one of the fairest and most conscientious legal members that I was privileged to work with, had a strong letter published in the Melbourne *Age*. I too was angry over some comments made by conservative politicians and sent the following letter to *The Age* which was also published:

The Editor,

In the furore triggered by the new appointments made by Attorney General George Brandis to the Federal AAT and the ill-judged criticisms of the AAT by Minister Peter Dutton, important aspects have been overlooked. Members of the AAT are not free to make any decision they please but are obliged to weigh evidence presented by the appellant and the relevant government department and then decide the matter according to the law. If a government department or relevant minister is unhappy with a decision, it can be appealed to the Federal Court and if need be, the High Court. The fact that many decisions deemed by ministers to be unsatisfactory have not been appealed suggests that the government department accepted that each decision was correct under the relevant law. If decisions are consistent with the law but are truly unsatisfactory or unfair, the minister can seek to change the law via Parliament. This is not unusual and is at times influenced by cases reviewed by a higher court.

Attempts to stack the AAT are regrettable, especially when competent hard-working members are not re-appointed. Such attempts are also ineffective because the new members are obliged to base their decisions on the evidence and the law.

Two AAT cases particularly come to mind whenever I think about the role that medical members can play. One involved a man who had served in the Navy and was seeking compensation for post-traumatic stress disorder. He claimed he had gone through a series of traumatic events including the Voyager disaster* and the collapse of the Westgate Bridge in Melbourne† but his naval records and the timing of these events strongly indicated that these claims were not true. He had been assessed by four independent psychiatrists over some years and none had raised any concerns about his accounts. Quite late in the AAT hearing, I suddenly sensed the reason for the mounting discrepancies between his strong

---

* This was a major Australian naval peacetime disaster in 1964 involving a collision between the destroyer, HMAS *Voyager*, and the aircraft carrier, HMAS *Melbourne*.
† In 1970 during its construction, a span of the Westgate Bridge in Melbourne collapsed killing many workers.

beliefs and the naval and other records – he almost certainly was a man with the condition of pseudologia fantastica.[*] This possibility was supported by the final expert witness to give evidence, an experienced psychiatrist who by chance was very familiar with this unusual condition, when all the relevant material was placed before him.[†] The Tribunal dismissed his claim.

The second case was equally unusual. A man was appealing against a decision to deny him compensation for a work-related injury. He too had seen a number of psychiatrists. When he gave evidence, he described his visit to see the first of these psychiatrists. He seemed unhappy with something about that visit so I asked him to describe the attendance in detail. He recalled that he attended the psychiatrist in an old house in an inner Melbourne suburb where the doctor practised. He sat in a corridor and the

[*] Pseudologia fantastica was first described in the German literature in 1891 and, as the name implies, refers to people who tell false stories about themselves. No single internationally agreed definition for this uncommon entity exists. Neither is it agreed that it is an entity in its own right as some writers have depicted it as part of a wider spectrum of human behaviour that incorporates the entities of the Munchausen syndrome (factitious disorder) and pathological lying. However, there is general agreement that the key features of pseudologia fantastica are: (a) the stories told are not entirely improbable and are built on a matrix of partial truth; (b) the stories are enduring for that person; (c) the stories are told for self-aggrandisement rather than for personal profit; (d) the stories are distinguishable from delusions in that the teller insists on them being true even when confronted with objective evidence of the real facts; and (e) the storyteller's motivations seem to be internal rather than external. King, B H and Ford, C V, 'Pseudologia fantastica', *Acta Psychiatr. Scand*, vol. 77, 1988, 1–6.

[†] Watson and Repatriation Commission [2010] AATA 220; 29 March 2010. http://www.austlii.edu.au/cgi-bin/viewdoc/au/cases/cth/AATA/2010/220.html.

doctor came to give him a detailed questionnaire to fill in. He took it home and mailed it back to the doctor. He never saw the psychiatrist again and never had a psychiatric history taken by that doctor. The man's wife who was with him at the 'consultation' supported her husband's evidence. From the answers to the questionnaire, the psychiatrist constructed a detailed report which read as though a proper consultation had taken place. This unprofessional conduct had serious repercussions as his report was inaccurate in several aspects and yet had subsequently been accepted by other psychiatrists who had drawn wrong conclusions because of the inaccuracies. With the support of the AAT member in charge of that hearing, the psychiatrist's conduct was notified to the Medical Board. I learned much later that he had been the subject of an informal hearing by a panel of the Board and was reprimanded. I felt that he was very lucky to receive such a minor penalty. It seemed to me that the panel had overlooked the fact that the medical report for which he was paid represented a form of fraud.[‡]

A no-fault medical negligence scheme

On a different topic, the adversarial system we have in Australia for determining if damages are to be paid to patients harmed through medical negligence has often been criticised but no government in recent times has had the courage to deal with the vested interests at work. As a system, it can be very slow, very expensive, very stressful for all parties, unfair to many who seek compensation, and

‡ Butterfield and the Repatriation Commission [2009] AATA 609. http://www.austlii.edu.au/cgi-bin/viewdoc/au/cases/cth/AATA/2009/609.html.

inimical to the concept of full and prompt reporting and open disclosure of adverse events. As one US commentator has described them, court cases over medical negligence involving competing hired medical experts can be regarded as a 'contest of liars'. I believe that changing to a no-fault compensation system would bring enormous advantages by correcting many of these problems.

Very few doctors will be aware that at about the same time that our near neighbour, New Zealand, introduced a 'no-fault' system of dealing with medical injury, Australia too was on the brink of doing the same. The Whitlam ALP government had legislation ready to be introduced when Whitlam was famously dismissed in 1975. Now many countries have such schemes, including Sweden, Finland, Norway, Denmark, France, New Zealand, and some US states.

In response to an alarming report on adverse events in our hospitals, the federal government established the Australian Commission for Safety and Quality in Health Care (ACSQHC). Its activities have focussed especially on system-related adverse events such as medication errors, operations on the wrong body part and prevention of in-hospital falls, as well as promoting the concept of 'open disclosure'. Open disclosure after an adverse event is defined as saying sorry and giving a factual explanation of what happened, the consequences of the adverse event, and steps required to manage the event and prevent recurrence. Encouraging discussion of the facts without attributing blame is said to not represent an admission of liability. Indeed, all Australian states and territories have passed legislation to make it clear that saying sorry cannot be used in civil action as an admission of liability.

However, doctors remain fearful of being sued and worried about the implications of saying sorry, claiming, not unreasonably, that there is a fine line between expressing regret and admitting liability. In addition to this concern, there are a number of barriers to the widespread use of the open disclosure approach, including lack of promulgation and education, unwillingness to admit error, and uncertainty as to what or how much to disclose. An environment of naming and shaming of doctors remains a problem. Medical students are taught about new approaches to patient safety and reporting near misses but then observe quite different behaviours on the part of their role models.

There is an additional concern with the ACSQHC concept of open disclosure which to my knowledge has not been voiced. As I read the detailed document on open disclosure, I sense that one of its major aims is to reduce the risk of hospitals being sued. If I am correct, this then creates the ethical dilemma of possibly denying financial or other assistance to patients who have been injured by medical treatment. Persons injured through health care are more likely to sue for damages if they feel that their concerns have been ignored or if they have not been communicated with appropriately. Complete open disclosure should also address their rights to compensation.

In collaboration with a lawyer colleague, Professor David Weisbrot, we have campaigned to push for a no-fault indemnity scheme,* so far without success. At the national level, the idea was briefly canvassed in the report

* Weisbrot, D, Breen, K J, 'A no-fault compensation system for medical injury is long overdue', *Medical Journal of Australia*, 2012, 197: 296–

of the Productivity Commission on the National Disability Scheme a few years back but put on the 'back burner'. There is perhaps more likelihood of Victoria going it alone with a no-fault system as a report prepared for government by Stephen Duckett in October 2016 entitled *Targeting Zero: supporting the Victorian hospital system to eliminate avoidable harm and strengthen quality of care* recommended this reform. There are very strong vested interests in the legal profession and in sections of the medical profession that would prefer to see the inequitable but lucrative adversarial system continue, so I am not holding my breath.

The euthanasia debate

Like many doctors, I observed the Victorian debate around the subject of euthanasia (now called medically assisted dying, a term George Orwell might have been proud to invent) with some dismay. While I am prepared to accept the will of the people if assisted dying is made legal, I am fiercely opposed to handing this assisting role to doctors. It is contrary to all the caring principles that medicine has stood for over centuries. Should it become law, then I would wish to see the authority to prescribe death to be limited to a small number of doctors, allowing patients to continue to have complete confidence in the bulk of the medical profession. My views are summarised in the following letter sent to the Editor of *The Age* in July 2016. Not all the letter was

8; Breen, K J, Weisbrot, D, 'Medical negligence system must change', *Medical Journal of Australia* 2015, 202: 574–5, and Weisbrot, D, Breen, K J, 'Why don't we create a no-fault scheme for medical injuries?', http://theconversation.com/why-dont-we-create-a-no-fault-scheme-for-medical-injuries-25329.

published and the omitted segments have been bracketed.

To the Editor

If Victorians decide to legalise euthanasia [(physician-assisted suicide)], one hopes that it will be a decision based on careful debate and not on sensationalised declarations of need from a minority of doctors. The community might then have a better chance of understanding why the majority of doctors continue to oppose legalisation, opposition based on factors including the rarity of requests from patients receiving good palliative care, the possibility that requests are driven by distressed relatives and not the patient, the difficulty in drawing up laws that adequately protect vulnerable people who they feel they are a burden to society, and the undermining of trust in doctors generally if some participate in physician-assisted suicide.

[The community could also be correctly informed of the rapid development of tolerance to morphine (increasing doses required to maintain symptom control) and not misinterpret this as a deliberate method of hastening death. When morphine is used appropriately and skilfully, there is no evidence that it hastens or causes death.]

Should legalisation become a reality, it will be preferable that assistance be provided by persons other than doctors, or by a small number of clearly identified doctors, so that trust in doctors generally is not undermined. Involving doctors seeks to legitimise as a medical process what is really a social and legal intervention.

I have been concerned about several aspects of how assisted dying has been dealt with by the media but the aspect that has upset me the most has been what appears to me to be either deliberate misunderstanding or gross ignorance of the response of the human body to pain killing and sedating

239

drugs such as morphine. It is well established that tolerance to these drugs develops quite quickly. Tolerance means that the body adapts to the drug and as a result, increased doses are needed to achieve the same degree of pain relief and sedation. If this scientific fact is ignored, it becomes very easy to portray doctors who carefully increase morphine doses over time as engaging in mercy killing. I suggest that fear of being so portrayed has influenced the professional practice of many doctors, especially less experienced ones, so that patients with terminal illnesses are indeed now often under treated. Closely related to my views on this topic is the oft repeated observation of experienced doctors that the judicious use of morphine can prolong patients' lives, not shorten them, especially where a desire to be present for a significant family event is driving a will to live. The views of doctors are readily ignored in an era of alternative facts and denial of professional expertise and experience. More sadly, I was on the losing side of this debate as legislation authorising medically-assisted dying passed both Houses of Parliament in Victoria in November 2017.

Is the medical profession at risk of being over-regulated?

Over-regulation of the medical profession is another issue of concern. The badly designed national registration scheme has exaggerated the problem and while the national system continues, I remain pessimistic for the quality of the lives of Australia's doctors who are mostly caring, competent and striving to do their best. Nothing exemplifies over-regulation better than the push by the

Medical Board of Australia to introduce the UK General Medical Council process of revalidation. There is zero evidence that revalidation produces more caring or more competent doctors. More importantly, the system takes doctors away from their patients and costs the health care system money. As recently as September 2017, the president of the GMC described the 'simple' burden of revalidation thus: 'The GMC simply requires, over a five-year period, one collection of colleague feedback; annual whole practice appraisal; evidence of quality improvement or audit activity; a discussion of any complaints and compliments; and a self-declaration of health'.* To describe this as a simple burden is laughable.

It seems that some leaders of the medical profession in Australia wish to embrace this unproven scheme without consulting the profession at large and without considering the cost implications or the likelihood that many doctors will pay lip service to the process. To add this extra layer of regulation on top of a longstanding requirement for Australian doctors to engage in approved continuing education programs seems to me to be an enormous folly.† Happily, in November 2017, the Medical Board announced that it would not proceed with a UK-style revalidation process. Instead the Board proposes to strengthen its requirements for continuing professional development (CPD) and plans a system of regular health checks for doctors over the age of seventy.‡

---

* Stephenson, T, 'On revalidation the GMC is listening to you', *BMJ*, 2017, 358: j4215.

† Breen, K J, 'Revalidation – what is the problem and what are the possible solutions?', *Medical Journal of Australia*, 2014, 200: 153–6.

‡ http://www.medicalboard.gov.au/News/2017-11-28-media-re-

I am not convinced that adding to the current CPD requirements has an adequate evidence base. My view is shared by experienced colleagues and together we have argued publicly that further thought and wide debate about the Medical Board's proposals is needed. We would like to see doctors provided with alternative paths to satisfy the Medical Board of their continuing competence and safety to practise. We also believe that CPD needs to be reformed and have urged weaning CPD from drug company funding as well as suggesting that all CPD programs need to have definite aims and a clearly stated curriculum.*

There are challenges ahead for the medical profession but perhaps it was always thus. The fragmentation of the profession into multiple specialties makes it much more difficult to develop a unified view on many of these challenges. Governments, federal and state, see the Australian Medical Association as the formal source of the views of the profession. This may have been appropriate in the distant past but now may be unwise as the proportion of doctors who are members of the AMA is believed to be well under 50%.

The challenges ahead

Of the challenges facing the profession, the ones that I am most passionate about are securing adequate funding for truly comprehensive doctors health programs; doing away

lease-professional-performance-framework.aspx.
* Breen, K, Whelan, G and Watson, K. Compulsory continuing professional development for doctors needs a rethink. https://croakey.org/changes-to-continuing-professional-development-requirements-for-doctors-need-a-rethink/.

with mandatory reporting of ill-health by treating doctors; and changing the medical negligence system to a no-fault scheme. The Victorian Doctors Health Program is adequately funded for the moment but its future is still not fully secure. Perhaps new leadership of the Medical Board of Australia will be required for this to happen. The health ministers have agreed to a new approach to mandatory reporting but how long this will take to deliver and what it will look like is anyone's guess.

I suggest that the best chance of moving to a no-fault medical indemnity scheme lies with the Victorian Government. Victoria has a proud history of being the first jurisdiction to introduce many vital social reforms such as compulsory seat belt legislation and breath-testing drivers for alcohol. Victorians are familiar with no-fault insurance systems for motor vehicle accidents and for work-related injuries. Creating a no-fault medical indemnity system is a complex task and is likely to be simpler to pioneer at a state level than nationally. The strongly opposed forces which include law firms for whom medical negligence is their 'bread and butter', and the multiple doctors who also depend on the adversarial system, might be easier to stare down in a single jurisdiction.

The predicted benefits of such a change are enormous. They include for patients a quicker, fairer and more just access to help after a medical injury. For doctors, there will be no less accountability but the destruction of morale and careers that at times result from the adversarial system will disappear. There will be savings from far less spending on lawyers and court actions which can be redirected to where the money is needed. There will be the opportunity for far more effective reporting (and acting on) near misses and adverse events, and for open disclosure to become truly routine. Depending upon the design of the scheme, it should cost the community and the medical profession less than the current medical indemnity system. The design can be informed through the decades of experience of several developed nations. All that is needed is an imaginative and courageous minister of health for this to happen. My wish is that it happens in my life time.

Epilogue

My aims in writing this account were several. They included setting the record straight about my lack of formal training in medical ethics, seeking to encourage all doctors to feel confident about participating in debates involving medical ethics, and providing insights into aspects of the work of several agencies that influence the conduct of doctors, especially medical boards. An alternate title for this story could have been the 'diary of a medical regulator', but medical regulator is a term that is not presently popular with the medical profession.

My account should confirm that I am not an ethicist, if one uses that term to describe a person professionally educated, trained and qualified in some aspect of ethics. A more accurate self-description might be that I am a physician who was given the opportunity to learn much about medical regulation, medical ethics and medical professionalism and that I have used this opportunity to share as widely as possible the lessons that I learnt. My early experience on the Medical Board of Victoria convinced me that most doctors generally seek to do the right thing, despite at times rendering some patients very angry, and that with access to only a little more knowledge of the core elements of what is required to be a good doctor, they are very unlikely to come before the Medical Board again. My early belief in this regard has been backed up by recent research that shows that only a small cohort of 'recidivist' doctors are the cause of a large proportion of the complaints made to the Medical Board.*

It remains to be seen if my efforts will result in more medical colleagues becoming comfortable with discussing ethical issues as they arise in daily practice. If any doctor seeks to compartmentalise 'ethics' as something done elsewhere by trained ethicists, then I will have failed comprehensively. If on the other hand, competent and caring doctors appreciate that they are teaching ethical behaviour through the role-modelling for, and mentoring of, medical students and junior doctors, and if they also appreciate that medical professionalism is a global term that describes how they should go about being good doctors who always put the interests of their patients first, then they are well on the way to being equipped to discuss 'medical ethics' with anyone. In my view 'professionalism' is a quality very much based on the ethical and legal principles that underpin good medical practice. Through understanding professionalism as it is presently taught and demonstrating professionalism consistently through their approach to patients, doctors can be comfortable that they are ethically competent even though they may have had little formal education in medical ethics.

My account may have also given you more insight into the problems that a small proportion of doctors can create through serious and sometimes repeated unprofessional conduct in clinical practice or through misconduct in medical

* Bismark M M, Spittal M J, Gurrin L C, et al., 'Identification of doctors at risk of recurrent complaints: a national study of health-care complaints in Australia', *BMJ Qual Saf*, vol. 22, 2013: 532–40.

research, and why these behaviours can be so harmful. These behaviours also sully the reputation of the vast majority of doctors who strive to do the best they can, sometimes in very challenging situations. Perhaps you also now know more about doctors' health services and why these are vital, why sexual misconduct is always harmful, and why most doctors deny the influence of drug companies on their prescribing behaviour. You might even be convinced that a no-fault medical indemnity system, when it is introduced, will bring benefits for the community as well as for the medical profession. You might also sense that medicine is now at risk of being over-regulated.

My account has necessarily covered a significant of part of the second half of my professional career, a time spent, mostly by accident and not by design, working in a number of agencies that help to guide the medical profession and protect the public. If you have found the account interesting and have learned a little from it, I will be well satisfied.

INDEX

About the Author

Dr Kerry John Breen, AM, MBBS, MD, FRACP graduated from the University of Melbourne in 1964 and trained as a physician, specialising in gastroenterology. He was the inaugural Director of the Gastroenterology Department at St Vincent's Hospital, Melbourne (1978–93), at which hospital at various times he also held academic, general medical and management positions. He served as President of the Medical Practitioners Board of Victoria (1994–2000) and as President of the Australian Medical Council (1997–2000). He served as Chair of the Australian Health Ethics Committee of the National Health and Medical Research Council (2000–6) and as NHMRC Commissioner of Complaints (2007–13). He also served as Chairman of the Board of the Victorian Doctors Health Program (2005–9). From 2006 to 2014, he was a part-time member of the Federal Administrative Appeals Tribunal. He is currently a member of the Australian Research Integrity Committee and holds an appointment as an Adjunct Professor in the Department of Forensic Medicine at Monash University. In 2007 he was made a Member of the Order of Australia for 'For service to medicine through the advancement of medical ethics and professional standards of training and practice and to the specialty of gastroenterology as a clinician and teacher'.

He has published over 120 peer reviewed academic papers as well as several opinion pieces for the print media and internet publications. He is the lead author of *Good Medical Practice: Professionalism Ethics and Law* (4th edn.), published in 2016 by the Australian Medical Council and the sole author of *So You Want to be a Doctor: A Guide for Prospective Medical Students in Australia* published by the Australian Council for Educational Research in 2012. His biography of the late Professor Carl de Gruchy, entitled *The Man We Never Knew: Carl de Gruchy Medical Pioneer*, will be published by the Faculty of Medicine at the University of Melbourne later this year.

9 781925 801224